Ricardo Alencar Libório

Diagnosis of zoonoses in production animals in the state of Tocantins

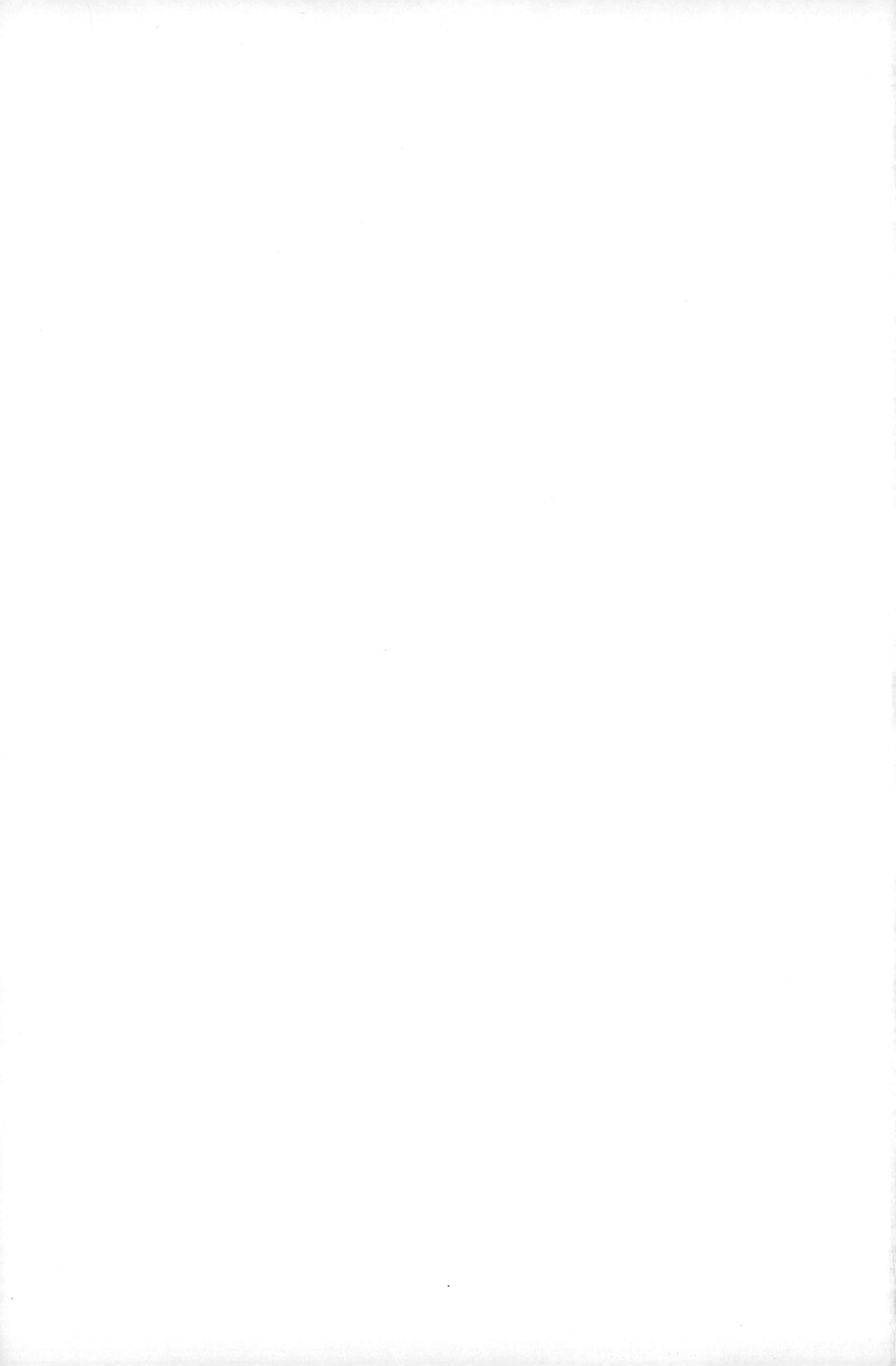

Ricardo Alencar Libório

Diagnosis of zoonoses in production animals in the state of Tocantins

Diagnosis of zoonoses caused by nematodes, trematodes and cestodes in production animals in the state of Tocantins

Imprint

Any brand names and product names mentioned in this book are subject to trademark, brand or patent protection and are trademarks or registered trademarks of their respective holders. The use of brand names, product names, common names, trade names, product descriptions etc. even without a particular marking in this work is in no way to be construed to mean that such names may be regarded as unrestricted in respect of trademark and brand protection legislation and could thus be used by anyone.

Cover image: www.ingimage.com

This book is a translation from the original published under ISBN 978-613-9-62490-4.

Publisher:
Sciencia Scripts
is a trademark of
Dodo Books Indian Ocean Ltd. and OmniScriptum S.R.L publishing group

120 High Road, East Finchley, London, N2 9ED, United Kingdom
Str. Armeneasca 28/1, office 1, Chisinau MD-2012, Republic of Moldova, Europe
Printed at: see last page
ISBN: 978-620-7-72809-1

SUMMARY

I dedicate this victory especially to God, for giving me strength and courage at every moment of my life. To my parents, for their trust, patience, love and support in making this dream come true. To all my family and friends who have always helped me, directly or indirectly.

ACKNOWLEDGMENTS

First of all, I thank God for granting me this grace and for always being present in my life, giving me health, protection, peace, love, strength, wisdom and perseverance.

To my parents, Helvécio and Eleuda, for their love, affection, attention, support and trust in me.

To my brother Francisco Libório and my sisters Vera Lùcia and Maria do Carmo, who supported me at all times.

To my nephews Victor Eduardo and Polyanna, for their love and affection. To my beloved niece Ana Izabel *(in memorian),* for her eternal tenderness.

To all the friends who helped me make this dream come true, for their prayers, advice and, above all, for their affection, my sincere thanks.

To the teachers at UFT - School of Veterinary Medicine and Zootechny, who were essential to my professional development. I would especially like to thank those who, in addition to their teaching, gave me their friendship.

To my friends and colleagues from the Master's and Doctorate courses, for the time spent together, the teachings, the moments of joy, the difficulties and the friendship shared.

To all the staff at the School of Veterinary Medicine and Zootechny, especially the postgraduate secretaries, colleagues linked to the Fênix company and other collaborators for their attention and friendship.

To the Parasitology study group at the UFT School of Veterinary Medicine and Zootechny, especially Professor Dr. Marcello Sato, Dr. Megumi Sato, Francisco Farias, Camila, Fernanda, Eduardo, Ronaldo and the other colleagues and professors who encouraged me throughout this period.

To the directors of Frigorificos Boi Forte (Araguaina) and Boi Brasil (Alvorada), to Veterinarians Dagoberto Machado Prata, Zuley Ferreira Pontes *(in memorian)* and Frédson Ronei Càndido, from SIF - 723 and to Veterinarians Toscano Correia Castro and José Josivaldo Antunes, from SIF - 1723 for their support and teachings.

To the staff of SIF's 723 and 1723, especially Mr. Josemar, Mr. Garcia, Mr. Ézio and Mr. Parriao, for their friendship, attention and support, and to the other employees of these industries for their collaboration and support.

To the owners of Made-Mar fishmongers, for their attention and support in carrying out this research.

To the National Council for Scientific and Technological Development (CNPq) for its financial support in carrying out this research.

1   GENERAL INTRODUCTION

It is estimated that the national cattle herd has around 177.7 million animals. Internationally, Brazil has become one of the largest suppliers of meat, with more than 7.8 million tons of carcass equivalent, and it could certainly become the largest supplier due to its high production potential. With regard to the state of Tocantins, beef cattle farming deserves to be highlighted, as it has a cattle herd of around 6.9 million head and plays a significant role in shaping the gross domestic product, making it one of the most important agribusiness sectors in the national economy (ANUALPEC, 2010).

Parasitology is an important branch of zoology that studies the diversity of relationships between parasites and their hosts. In this context, parasitology is increasingly an intercurricular activity, involving various medical and public health disciplines (REY, 2008).

There are various tools used in parasitology studies, from classic techniques to modern forms of diagnosis, using molecular biology. To this end, it is necessary to know the parasite-host relationship, as well as their interrelationships, due to the large number of zoonoses that can be caused, given the biological cycle of the parasite under study, in addition to the soil and climate conditions for its development (URQUHART et al., 2008).

Several factors play a role in the geographical distribution of parasitic diseases, such as the presence of suitable susceptible hosts, human migrations, favorable environmental conditions and high biotic potentials.

Zoonoses caused by parasites cause serious economic damage and interfere with animal production, as well as causing carcasses and viscera to be condemned in slaughterhouses. Notification of the occurrence of certain diseases such as cysticercosis in cattle, for example, is mandatory and must be carried out routinely by veterinarians and slaughter technicians in establishments with state or federal inspections (REZENDE, 2006).

The implications of these organisms for public health are also noteworthy, since emerging zoonoses caused by mammalian parasite larvae present in the soil and aquatic environment have been acquiring great medical importance in the human population (REY, 2008).

Therefore, studies that address the different classes of nematode, cestode and trematode helminths are necessary in order to gain a better understanding of the epidemiological chain, helping with prevention, treatment and diagnosis of these parasites, providing animal health welfare and avoiding economic losses in the production chain.

Therefore, this study evaluated the zoonoses caused by Nematodes (*Onchocerca* spp.), Cestodes (*Taenia* spp.) and Trematodes (Heterophyideos), in different animal species and in different ecosystems. In addition, emphasis will be placed on each of these classes of parasites, with a view to gaining a better understanding of each of them.

2 LITERATURE REVIEW

2.1 CLASS NEMATODA

Nematodes are commonly called cylindrical worms because of their appearance in cross-section. They are distributed in ten superfamilies, among which are nematodes of veterinary importance, including the Filarioidea, whose main representatives are the following nematodes: *Dirofilaria, Onchocerca* and *Parafilaria. The* typical features of these nematodes are their slender, long bodies, their indirect evolutionary cycle and their infection by insect L3 (infective larva) (URQUHART, 2008).

The effects of nematodes on cattle depend on the species and the degree of infection. However, in extensive beef cattle farms in Central Brazil, mortality is low and verminosis mainly contributes to the animals' low growth rate (BIANCHIN, 1979).

However, within the superfamily Filarioidea, there are differences in biological behavior, since the most primitive forms lay eggs (they are viable for vectors in dermal exudates) and the most highly evolved forms lay larvae, called microfilariae (the first larval form of filarid worms), as occurs with *Onchocerca* spp. (URQUHART, 2008).

2.1.1 Onchocerciasis in animals

Onchocerciasis is a disease caused by parasitic nematodes of the genus *Onchocerca* spp. The disease is transmitted by dipterans of the family Simuliidae of the genus *Simulium* spp. commonly known as the mosquito borrachudo or pium, and can cause blindness in its acute stage. Originally from the African continent, where it is widespread, this disease was discovered in Latin America and Guatemala in 1917, with subsequent records in Mexico, Venezuela, Colombia and Brazil (OGBOGU, 1990). The species of the genus *Onchocerca* spp. are generally specific parasites of ungulates and humans, parasitizing their hosts for several years (WILDENBURG et al, 1997).

Of this genus, seven species have been described as parasitizing cattle: *Onchocerca gutturosa, O. gibsoni, O. lienalis, O. dukei, O. armillata, O. ochengi* and *O. stilesi,* the first three being the most described in the world literature (PAIVA et al, 1984).

Most species of *Onchocerca* spp. are generally of low pathogenicity and, consequently, of little interest in veterinary medicine, but there has been an increase in the frequency of transmission to humans (TRESS et al. 1992; TRESS et al. 2000).

According to Wildenburg et al (1997), the pathogenicity of filarid infection in humans and cattle has been observed with the presence of an allergic reaction in the host as well as the presence of microfilariae in the subcutaneous tissue. Bovine *onchocerciasis* is caused by several species of parasites of the genus *Onchocerca* spp. The adult worms and larvae live in the connective tissue, and the larvae, the microfilariae, are dermatotrophic. There is a diversity of species of *Onchocerca* spp. described, but the greatest difficulty is in recovering the intact form of the parasites in adult form for their morphological study, as they can be in different locations, making it difficult to study and identify these helminths.

According to Bevilaqua and Dorchies (1999a), the prevalence of onchocerciasis in temperate countries is lower than in tropical countries, probably due to seasonal transmission. In studies on the parasite in France, it was observed that parasitism is highest in spring and summer.

The age of the cattle does not play a predominant role in determining infection because its effect is only significant when associated with the seasons. On the other hand, the seasons are a determining factor in the prevalence and intensity of infection (GUDERIAN et al., 1992).

The pre-patent period for *Onchocerca gutturosa* is approximately seven months. The presence of this parasite has been observed in animals aged between three and four years, up to seven years old, confirming that age is not significant for the presence of infection by this parasite (BEVILAQUA; DORCHIES, 1999b).

According to Beytut et al. (2005), in Europe the two most abundant species of *Onchocerca* spp. that parasitize cattle are *O. lienalis* and *O. gutturosa*, which are distributed all over the world. *O. gutturosa* lives in the loose connective tissue of the cervical ligament and other tendons, while *O. lienalis and O. gutturosa* live in the cervical ligament and other tendons.

lienalis lives in the gastrosplenic region of the peritoneal cavity. The microfilariae of both are found in the umbilical region, which is a favorite location for these parasites.

The microfilariae of *O. gutturosa* are about 270 µm (micrometers) long and 3-5 µm wide, while those of *O. iienalis* are 236 µm long and 5-7 µm wide. The parasitic lesions found are generally diagnosed in the tendons, ligaments and fasciae of the hind legs, indicating infestation by *O. gutturosa,* which predominates in these places (BEYTUT et al., 2005).

Another common helminth in cattle is *Onchocerca iienalis, which is* usually found in cattle raised in temperate climates, where thousands of microfilariae can be extracted from the skin of these animals after they have been slaughtered in slaughterhouses. The infective larvae (L3) can be produced through the cultivation of *Simulium* spp. vectors, which has allowed studies of the dynamics of the antibody response after experimental infection (SANTIN-DURAN et al., 1979).

The presence of *Onchocerca* spp. in cattle is considered common in Finland, but it has been proven that the amount of pathological changes and the condemnation of infected parts is very low in relation to the prevalence of microfilariae that were found in the samples analyzed (SOLISMAA et al., 2008).

Onchocerca spp. are generally considered to be of low pathogenicity to cattle and therefore of little veterinary interest. The pathological lesions that occur on cattle carcasses are mild and infrequent, and most of them escape the eyes of meat inspectors at slaughterhouses. In this sense, it is difficult to assess the situation of onchocerciasis and the economic losses it can cause, but it is important to raise awareness of its existence so that it can be controlled and public health policies developed (DOHNAL et al., 1990).

Mark (1979), in studies on the occurrence of *Onchocerca* spp. in cattle in the United States, reported the presence of *Onchocerca gutturosa and O. lienalis* in cattle. There is some controversy about the exact taxonomic classification of these parasites. This can be attributed to several factors, including, above all, the lack of agreement on the morphological criteria useful in identifying species and poor morphological descriptions of the species already described.

2.2 CESTODA CLASS

The class Cestoidea (= Cestoda) comprises animals with a body (strobilus) that is generally ribbon-shaped, segmented and previously provided with an attachment organ (scolex), with adhesive structures of various types, each segment containing one and sometimes two sets of male and female reproductive organs (REY, 2008).

Almost all cestodes of veterinary importance are in the order Cyclophyllidea, the two exceptions being in the order Pseudophyllidea. The cestodes most frequently found parasitizing humans are cosmopolitan cyclophiles, such as *Taenia solium, Taenia saginata, Echinococcus granulosus* and *Hymenolepis nana*; rarely others (REY, 2008).

However, this class is represented as follows: *Taeniidae* family (Genera - *Echinococcus granulosus, Taenia solium* and *Taenia saginata*); *Hymenolepididae* family (Genera - *Hymenolepis nana, Humenolepis diminuta*); *Dilepididae* family (Genus - *Dipylidium caninum*) and *Diphyllobotridae* family (Genera - *Diphyllobothrium latum and Spirometra*) (URQUHART et al., 2008).

The present experiment refers mainly to the *Taeniidae* family, genus *Taenia* spp., as it is the most important genus, both the adult and larval stages being important in human health and veterinary medicine. The main species studied was *Taenia saginata,* because the intermediate stage of this cestode is found in the muscles of cattle and often poses economic problems for the meat industry and constitutes a public health risk (URQUHART et al., 2008).

As a public health problem, cysticercosis cannot be ignored by public inspection bodies and consumers (UNGAR and GERMANO, 1992).

Currently, there are believed to be 77 million people parasitized by *Taenia saginata* in the world, of which 32 million are in Africa, 11 million in Asia, two million in South America and one million in North America (SILVA, 2005). There are three stages to the parasite population: adult in the definitive host, eggs in the environment and cysticercus (larval stage) in the intermediate host (GEMMELL et al., 1983).

In some countries such as India, Africa, Mexico, Central and South America and in regions considered endemic such as North Korea, China, Indonesia, Southeast Asia and Eastern Europe, there is a high prevalence of this zoonosis (CARPIO, 2002; WHO, 2002; CDC, 2003). *Taenia saginata* is the most widespread parasite among those that cause *taeniasis* in men (CDC, 2003).

Teniasis is the disease caused by the adult stage of the parasite in the small intestine of humans. Cysticercosis is the disease caused by the parenteral metacestode stage in the tissues of humans and animals (SATO et al., 2004). Certainly, if humans are not infected with the parasite in the adult stage, this parasitic disease is rationally eradicable. Furthermore, if animals do not have access to human feces contaminated with parasite eggs, the life cycle cannot be completed (SCHANTZ et al., 1994).

However, cysticercosis is one of the parasitic diseases that deserve a lot of attention in our country, due to its high prevalence and the high socio-economic damage it causes. Data on bovine cysticercosis, an important zoonosis, is provided by the Federal Inspection Service (SIF), which obtains it through *post-mortem* inspections carried out by federal agricultural inspectors and their assistants on animals slaughtered in accredited slaughter establishments (SANTOS et al, 2004).

According to Monteiro et al, (2007), cysticercosis is a zoonosis caused by *Taenia saginata* larvae, from the ingestion of viable eggs present in the environment contaminated with human feces. *Taenia solium* also causes cysticercosis through the presence of its larvae in pork.

Man is the only definitive host of *T. saginata*. Intermediate hosts include cattle, buffalo, sheep, goats and reindeer. However, *Bos taurus indicus, B.taurus taurus* and *Bubalus bubalis* have the highest infection rates (CABARET et al, 2002).

One of the ways to prevent the spread of cysticercosis is through inspections of legal establishments. Raising awareness and improving the hygiene habits of the population, especially in rural areas, the effective fight against human teniasis, the fight against clandestine slaughterhouses and the notification of cases found are measures that contribute efficiently to the control, reduction of parasitism and sources of infection (MONTEIRO et al, 2007).

According to Monteiro et al, (2007), cysticercosis is a disease of cosmopolitan distribution and zoonotic character, of great importance in regions where the population has a low socioeconomic and cultural level, as it is believed that the highest incidence of cysticercosis occurs in places where sanitary conditions are poor, causing the teniasis/cysticercosis complex to take on an endemic character.

According to Urquhart et al. (2008), under natural conditions, the presence of cysticercus in bovine muscles is not associated with clinical symptoms, although experimentally, calves subjected to massive infection with *T. saginata* eggs have developed severe myocarditis and heart failure as a result of the development of cysticercus in the heart muscles.

2.2.1 EVOLUTIONARY CYCLE

According to Urquhart et al. (2008), the typical evolutionary cycle of these cestodes is indirect with an intermediate host. With few exceptions, the adult cestode is found in the small intestine of the definitive host, and the segments and eggs reach the outside through the feces.

When the egg is ingested by the intermediate host, gastric and intestinal secretions digest the embryophore and activate the oncosphere (hexacanth embryo - 6 hooks). Using its hooks, it lacerates the mucosa and reaches the blood or lymphatic circulation or, in the case of invertebrates, the body cavity (URQUHART et al., 2008).

Cysticercosis is caused by ingesting food or water contaminated with human feces containing *Taenia* eggs which, when they reach the stomach, are attacked by the digestive juices and hatch in the duodenum when they are stimulated by pancreatic juice (Figure 1). The free hexacanth embryo crosses the intestinal wall, enters the bloodstream and lodges in the tissues, mainly striated muscles (FORTES, 2004). There it develops into the larval stage (cysticercus), where it becomes infective in approximately 12 weeks (KASSAI, 1999).

The cysts measure 7 to 12 mm in length and 4 to 6 mm in width. The adult parasites (tapeworms) are specific to the definitive host, while the larval stages (cysticerci) are not specific to intermediate hosts (REY, 2008). Some authors maintain that human cysticercosis by *T. saginata* cysticerci is extremely rare or does not occur, but there is no scientific proof of this fact (SCHANTZ et al., 1994), while others admit the possibility of human cysticercosis by both species of tapeworm, precisely because of this lack of specificity of the larval stage for the intermediate host (REY, 2008).

Humans are the only definitive hosts of *Taenia saginata*. The adult worm, which is around 5 meters long, lives in the small intestine where it attaches itself by a structure called a scolex. They produce proglottids (each worm has 1,000 to 2,000 proglottids) which, if they become pregnant, detach from the worm and migrate to the anus or come out with the feces (about 6 per day). Each gravid proglottid contains between 80,000 and 100,000 eggs. The eggs can survive for months to years in the environment (CDC, 2003).

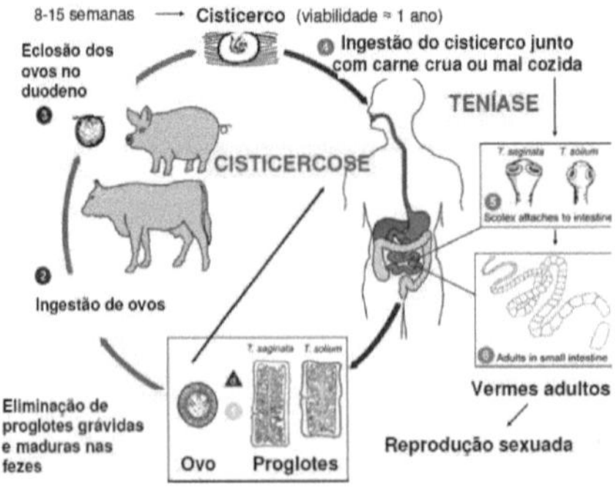

Figure 1 - Biological cycle of *Taenia* spp.

Source: CDC, 2003

According to Flisser et al. (2005), humans are the definitive hosts of *T. saginata* and are responsible for spreading the eggs in the environment. Generally, humans are contaminated by a single tapeworm (*T. saginata).* Contamination of livestock can occur through the ingestion of pasture, fodder or water contaminated with the parasite's eggs.

Humans become infected by eating raw or undercooked infected meat. The parasite develops in the small intestine, becoming sexually mature in approximately three months, where it begins to produce gravid proglottids, which are mobile and migrate to the host's anus spontaneously or are eliminated in the feces. In this way, the parasite can survive in the definitive host for several years. The presence of the tapeworm in the intestine can cause some symptoms in humans, such as diarrhea, weight loss and especially anal itching, caused by the migration of proglottids (FLISSER et al., 2005).

The ingestion of vegetation contaminated by the eggs (or proglottids) infects the intermediate host (cattle and other herbivores). In the animal's intestine, the eggs release the oncosphere, which evaporates, invades the intestinal wall and migrates to the striated muscles, where it develops into the cysticercus. The cysticercus can survive for many years in the animal. Ingestion of raw or undercooked meat with cysticercus infests humans. In the human intestine, the cysticercus develops 2 months later into an adult worm, which can survive for more than 30 years (CDC, 2003).

The adult form of the cestode parasite that causes cysticercosis, *Taenia saginata,* is present in the small intestine of humans. *Cysticercus bovis*, the larval form, occurs in the muscles of cattle. Both are from the Taenidae family, but they are two different stages in the parasite's biological cycle. Thus, in cattle, which are intermediate hosts of *T. saginata,* the disease is usually present without any clinical signs (UNGAR; GERMANO, 1992).

The spread of *T. saginata* is associated with the social, economic and cultural conditions of some populations in certain regions of the world. Another important factor in the spread of these diseases is the lack of a totally effective anthelmintic against the larval forms of these parasites, especially for the control of intermediate hosts (BIONDI et al., 2000).

The presence of viable *C. bovis* in bovine carcasses and viscera can cause infection in humans. Meat inspection in slaughterhouses, through post-mortem examination, is still the only practical way to detect and diagnose *C. bovis.* Worldwide, the biggest problems in controlling cysticercosis are related to the presence of cysticercus in animal tissues (DORNY; PRAET, 2007).

According to Dorny and Praet (2007), bovine cysticercosis caused by *Taenia saginata* is still present in Europe, causing major economic losses due to carcass condemnations, conditional utilization with cold treatment and the total downgrading of infected carcasses. The main reasons for the persistence of this zoonosis include the low sensitivity of current meat inspection protocols, the spread and survival of the eggs of these parasites in the environment, and extensive cattle breeding systems, which allow animals to drink water from streams. It is assumed that surface water and streams are potentially contaminated with *T. saginata* eggs.

2.2.2 DIAGNOSTIC METHODS

Currently, there are no proven resources for controlling cysticercosis *in vivo*. The most significant resource is the inspection of meat in a careful *post-mortem* examination and the evaluation of parasitized carcasses with adequate sanitation. Carcasses infected with cysticercus are investigated and their fate depends on the number of cysticercus found, and they can be frozen at -10°C for 15 days. However, in cases of infection with several cysts, the carcasses are evaluated and disposed of in accordance with legislation (SOUZA et al, 2007).

In Brazil, no laboratory diagnostic test is part of the health inspection routine, not even as a way of monitoring the accuracy and specificity of the macroscopic anatomopathological diagnoses made (COSTA, 2003). Identifying the infection in the animal depends on detailed inspection of the entire carcass during *post-mortem* examination. This technique identifies the carcass with massive or mild infection and serves as an early warning of the degree of contamination in a property or community (SOUZA et al, 2007).

According to Souza et al. (1978), knowledge of the location of the cysticercus is essential to improve the sensitivity of the inspection, since there is a lot of controversy between authors as to the organ with the highest concentration of cysts, which will increase the quality and reliability of *post-mortem* inspection in slaughterhouses.

Despite its limitations, inspection is still an important and specific method of identifying infection in animals. This technique identifies carcasses with massive and mild infections and serves as an early warning of the degree of infection on a farm or in a community. Criticism of the limitations of routine inspection is based on experimental work using slicing techniques, which are not routine in the inspection service, and the fact that this technique would make it impossible to market the meat (MINOZZO et al., 2002).

It's important to note that the presence of *C.bovis* in cattle carcasses can cause serious damage, from the producer to the meat-packing plant, and finally to the consumer, because when cysticercus is detected, the carcass can be used conditionally or even condemned completely. The industry incurs additional costs with the cold treatment of carcasses which, were it not for the presence of the disease, could have been sold immediately. Another important factor is the restrictions on exporting the meat, which in this case can only be destined for the domestic market. Producers, on the other hand, may receive nothing for their cattle if the carcass is totally condemned, or suffer a reduction in the amount paid by the industry in the case of partial condemnation (UNGAR et al., 1992).

The cysticercus is located in specific places in the animal and proper meat inspection is a practical way of detecting and diagnosing *Cysticercus bovis* (larval stage) of *Taenia saginata*. In this examination, incisions are made in the skeletal muscles and organs where cysticercuses are most frequently found and the diagnosis is made by visualizing them macroscopically. *Post-mortem* examination techniques for cattle were established in 1971 by the Ministry of Agriculture (FUKUDA et al, 1998).

Health inspection methods are standardized and are limited to the observation of organs, muscles and parts of the carcasses, which are considered to be the preferred location for the parasite, and as clandestine slaughter still exists in the country, it is believed that the occurrence of the disease is underestimated. Even so, cysticercosis has been the most frequently diagnosed pathology in *post-mortem* inspections carried out on cattle in slaughterhouses under Federal Inspection in Brazil (SILVA, 2005; REZENDE et al., 2006).

Furthermore, the fact that dead or calcified cysts are whitish in color and are easier to identify than live cysts, which are usually pale pink in color and can go unnoticed during inspection, should not be overlooked. It is therefore necessary to develop more effective and safer methods to improve the efficiency of diagnosis, especially the detection of cysticercosis in slaughterhouses (REZENDE et al., 2006).

Diagnostic methods have made great advances in recent years. The discovery of new methods in the field of molecular biology, such as the polymerase chain reaction (PCR), has direct application in the diagnosis of infectious and parasitic diseases (SINGH 1997).

The PCR technique has been one of the diagnostic methods used to identify teniasis and cysticercosis, as it does not require the integrity of the morphological structures to be maintained in order to identify and differentiate the parasite species involved in the teniasis/cysticercosis complex (SOMERS et al., 2006).

2.2.3 CONTROL AND PROPHYLAXIS

Taenia saginata and *Taenia solium* are agents that cause zoonoses because their life cycles depend on humans as the only definitive host. Their life cycles also depend on the relationship between humans and cattle (*T. saginata*) or pigs (*T. solium*). Interrupting the link between these hosts can result in the elimination of the parasite. Therefore, the control of teniasis/cysticercosis seems to be simple and easy (FLISSER et al., 2005).

Cysticercosis can be reduced when technological improvements are made on farms, such as the use of machinery in the formation and maintenance of pastures, where previously human labor was used. These factors possibly contribute to reducing the contamination of pastures by human feces (PIERRE, 2009).

The application of measures to control teniasis/cysticercosis depends on the epidemiological characteristics of the disease in the region, including economic, social and cultural conditions. The fundamental strategy is to interrupt the parasite's evolutionary cycle in order to prevent infection in animals and the human population (ORGANIZACION PANAMERICANA DE LA SALUD, 1994).

The strategies basically consist of: improving environmental sanitation conditions; treating the entire population; improving animal husbandry (avoiding animal access to human feces); increasing veterinary inspection of meat products; avoiding the slaughter and trade of clandestine products; health education emphasizing the adoption of hygiene habits (ORGANIZACION PANAMERICANA DE LA SALUD, 1994). For endemic countries, in addition to the measures mentioned above, measures could be adopted to freeze meat in order to reduce the transmission of the disease (PIERRE, 2009).

Based on the control measures indicated above, it is suggested that health education programs be implemented by local organizations so that the population freezes meat at temperatures below -15°C for at least 6 days. These measures could be taken at the slaughterhouse, even before the meat is distributed to the consumer market, thus reducing the transmission of the disease (FLISSER et al., 2005).

Preventive action against teniasis is based on a set of measures aimed at preventing human infection by *T. saginata* and thus interfering with the spread and blocking the cycle of this parasite in nature (SOUZA et al, 2007).

2.3 CLASS TREMATODA

The class Trematoda is divided into two main subclasses, the Monogenea, which has a direct evolutionary cycle, and the Digenea, which requires an intermediate host (URQUHART et al., 2008).

The representatives of the Monogenea subclass carry out their life cycle on just one host, and most of them parasitize marine and freshwater fish, although they can also parasitize amphibians, reptiles and molluscs. The Digenea subclass, on the other hand, has the largest number of parasites, and the life cycle of these trematodes involves between two and four hosts. Their main characteristic is that the primary host is always a vertebrate and any organ can be infected. Adult digenetic trematodes, commonly referred to as "leaf-shaped worms", occur mainly in the bile ducts, digestive tract and vascular system. They are generally dorso-ventrally flattened, have a blind digestive tract, attachment suckers and are hermaphroditic (THATCHER; NETO, 1994).

There are many families in the Trematoda class, and those that include parasites of great veterinary importance are *Fasciolidae, Dicrocoeliidae, Paramphistomatidae and Shistosomatidae. Of* lesser importance are *Troglotrematidae and Opisthorchiidae* (URQUHART et al., 2008).

Studies into the pathology and parasitology of fish are increasingly important in the context of fish farming worldwide. It seems inevitable that world populations will become increasingly dependent on artificial fish farming, while natural fish populations are gradually reduced by predatory fishing. As a result of these facts, artificial methods practiced in a semi-intensive way have come up against the scarcity of information on fish diseases, which in restrictive environments manifest themselves in a more vigorous and widespread way (THATCHER; NETO, 1994).

Parasitic zoonoses transmitted by fish are increasingly attracting the attention of researchers and health authorities around the world, due to the occurrence of public health problems in the population, which becomes infected through the consumption of raw or insufficiently cooked fish (OKUMURA et al., 1999).

Although zoonoses transmitted by trematodes through the consumption of fish cause liver diseases, which have been well documented in Vietnam, those that affect the intestine have an under-described occurrence. Recent research into the presence of metacercariae of human intestinal trematode parasites in fish caught and farmed in Vietnam has shown that there is a potential risk for communities that consume raw fish (DUNG et al., 2007).

According to Okumura et al. (1999), in Brazil there is a great demand for dishes made from raw fish, such as "sushi" and "sashimi", due to the influence of oriental cuisine today. In addition, there is data showing the presence of zoonotic parasites in Brazilian fish, both freshwater and saltwater. However, to date, there have been no reports of these parasites in humans in Brazil (with the exception of phagicolosis). It is believed that this is due to a lack of diagnosis, rather than the absence of these diseases in the country (DIAS et al., 1994).

Zoonoses transmissible by fish include anisakiasis, eustrongylidiasis, capillariasis, phagicolosis, clonorchiasis and diphyllobothriasis, among others. The main prevention measure is to abstain from eating raw or undercooked fish. It is also necessary to educate and raise awareness among the population, alerting them to the potential dangers of eating raw fish, as well as developing reliable techniques for inspecting and processing fish infected with parasites, in order to offer greater safety to the population (OKUMURA et al., 1999).

2.3.1 ZOONOSES CAUSED BY TREMATODES

Zoonoses caused by fish trematodes (Trematoda: Digenea) are of great importance to public health, with more than 50 million people affected worldwide, mainly in west and southwest Asia (SANTOS, 1995).

In Digenea, we find most of the fish parasites that have been described occurring in humans, including *Clonorchis sinensis, Opisthorchis viverrini, Opisthorchis felineus, Heterophyes* spp., *Metagonimus* spp, *Diplostomum spathaveum, Pygidiopsis summa, Stellantchasmus falcatus, Procerovum varium, Haplorchis* spp., *Nanophyetus schickhobalowi, Cryptocotyle lingua, Gonadosdasmius* spp., *Metorchis conjunctus, Echinoschasmus perfoliatus, Echinostoma hortense, Clinostomum complanatum, Pseudamphistomum truncatum* and *Isoparorchis hypselobagri.* (EIRAS, 1994b).

2.3.1.1 Fagicolosis

According to Castro (1994), infection by *Phagicola* spp. is relevant to public health, and due attention should also be paid to the damage this infection represents for animal production, which is another area of great responsibility for the veterinary surgeon.

The etiologic agent of phagicolosis, *Phagicola longa,* is a digenetic trematode belonging to the Heterophyidae family, which has a low parasite specificity, with many reports in the literature of different species of birds and mammals naturally parasitized by it. Thus, the great versatility of heterophyids in adapting to the intestines of different species of hosts, whether birds or mammals, gives them the possibility of also occurring in humans (BARROS et al, 1993).

Its distribution and epidemiology have been reported in several places on the American continent, including Brazil. The presence of *P. longa* metacercariae in all the fresh mullet specimens *(Mugil curema)* examined from the Patanemo Inlet in Venezuela was positive (CHIEFFI *et al.,* 1990).

According to Dias and Woiciechovskl (1994), the presence of this parasite was found in mugilids from the Cananéia and Registro regions (SP), with 100% prevalence in fish over 4 cm in total length. In samples of mugilid fish from the commercial fleet of the Baixada Santista (Santos and Guarujà - SP), the presence of encysted metacercariae of heterofiids, identified as *Phagicola longa,* was observed in 100% of these samples (ANTUNES; DIAS, 1994). According to CASTRO (1994), of the species of the genus *Phagicola* described in Brazil, *Phagicola longa* (also known as *P. longus),* has stood out among the others for being the only one, to date, capable of infecting man among other animals.

Infection by *Phagicola* spp. is a zoonosis that is still emerging and in need of study, particularly with regard to the parasite-host relationship. It is necessary for professionals involved in the study of zoonoses to carry out research aimed at investigating all the possible determinants related to its chain of transmission (CASTRO, 1994).

2.3.1.1.1 Phagicolosis in animals

According to Barros et al (1993), *P. longus is* host to piscivorous birds and mammals, causing pathological changes that tend to be subclinical and have a favorable prognosis. In an experimental study in which viable *P. longus* metacercariae were administered to a monkey (*Cebus apella*), it eliminated the parasites in its feces, demonstrating that this species is susceptible to infection by *Phagicola* spp. (CONROY, 1993; PEREZ, 1985).

2.3.1.1.2 Phagicolosis in humans

When man ingests the meat of a mullet infected with *Phagicola longus,* the parasite can develop and cause symptoms typical of parasitosis, such as colic, flatulence, diarrhea, weight loss and other conditions characteristic of verminosis in general (CHIEFFI et al., 1990).

Chieffi et al. (1990) reported the case of a patient with a history of eating raw fish prepared with mullet *(Mugil* spp.) in the region of Cananéia (SP). On physical examination, the patient complained of pain in the right lower quadrant and intestinal hypermotility. A stool test revealed the presence of *Phagicola* eggs (probably *P. longus),* with 120 eggs per gram of stool. The blood count showed slight eosinophilia and the patient was treated with praziquantel.

2.3.1.1.2.1 Prevention and control

Abstinence from eating raw or insufficiently cooked mullet meat is the main means of prevention (BARROS et al, 1993; CHIEFFI et al., 1990).

On the other hand, mullets refrigerated at 8°C in ice boxes pose a high risk to the human consumer, as they contain a large number of *P. longa* metacercariae, which are viable even after six days in refrigeration and can infect the final host when the product is prepared, if it is not processed properly. Metacercariae in mullet frozen at -2°C remain alive for approximately 12 hours. Heat treatment at 100°C for 30 minutes or 200°C for 15 minutes is enough to completely inactivate the metacercariae present in mullet *(Mugil curema)*. It is therefore recommended that consumers eat mullets well-cooked and not raw or semi-raw (SARAIVA, 1991).

2.3.2 CHLONORKYASE AND OPISTORKYASE

Clonorchiasis is a disease of the bile ducts caused by trematodes. *Opisthorchiasis* is a disease caused by small trematodes of cats and other piscivorous mammals, known as *Opisthorchis felineus.* The biology of these parasites, the characteristics of the disease and the control methods are essentially the same as those for clonorchiasis (BENESON, 1987).

The Opisthorchiidae (O. *felineus,* O. *viverrini* and *Clonorchis sinensis)* are the ones that cause the most severe consequences for humans and occur frequently in several Asian countries (EIRAS, 1994b).

Man is the most suitable definitive host for *C. sinensis* (EIRAS, 1994b). Reservoirs of the disease are humans, cats, dogs, pigs and other animals. The incubation period is undetermined and varies according to the number of parasites present. Parasitized individuals can expel viable eggs for 30 years, although there is no transmission between one person and another (BENESON, 1987).

2.3.2.1 Disease in humans and animals

According to Dias et al. (1994), the digenetic trematodes of the Heterophyidae family need fish as a second intermediate host in order to complete their biological cycle in birds and mammals. Laboratory studies, when started from infected molluscs, require fish species that are susceptible to infection by cercariae with the consequent formation of viable metacercariae. In these studies, the researchers recovered adult, ovigerous parasites from the small intestine of hamsters seven days after infection.

The symptoms of infections vary according to the species causing them. In any case, in the case of chronic liver infections, there may be damage to the bile ducts, gastrointestinal problems, jaundice, fatigue and cholangiocarcinoma (SANTOS, 1995). When the adult is located in the bile ducts, *C. sinensis* causes hyperplasia of the biliary epithelium, with subsequent dense pericanalicular fibrosis. The number of parasites can reach several thousand and practically all terminal bile ducts show fibrous thickening of the walls, with compression necrosis of the adjacent liver parenchyma

(FAUST et al., 1987).

2.3.2.2 Prevention and control

The most obvious way to avoid these parasites is to abstain from eating raw fish. However, ingrained cultural habits mean that reducing infection by this means is extremely unlikely, if not impossible. Prophylaxis consists of properly cooking all fish intended for human consumption, which will represent effective protection for the population (BENESON. 1987; FAUST et al., 1987).

It is also important to educate the population about the dangers of eating raw or improperly prepared fish and the need to dispose of feces correctly so as not to contaminate fish food sources, as well as prohibiting the use of human feces to fertilize fish ponds (BENESON. 1987; FAUST et al., 1987).

Well-established cultural and dietary traditions are extremely difficult to change, so available public health information combined with extensive treatment with praziquantel can effectively stop the consumption of raw fish, however long it may seem (SARAIVA, 1991).

As for prevention and control, according to Sato et al. (2009a) in studies in Thailand, they observed the occurrence of *Haplorchis taichui*, one of the most widespread intestinal digenetic trematodes in Southeast Asian countries. The metacercariae and the infective stage of the parasite have been found in many species of freshwater fish. Infection in humans occurs through the ingestion of contaminated raw or undercooked fish. *H. taichui* infections are generally asymptomatic, except in cases of severe parasitosis. For this reason, infections with *Haplorchis* spp. have been considered less important from a public health point of view.

Haplorchis taichui (Digenea: Heterophyidae) is one of the main and most common intestinal worms in humans, but little is known about the relationship between the number of eggs per gram of feces (OPG) and the actual parasite load in patients or the severity of the disease. In general, these parameters are good indicators for evaluating the effectiveness of anthelmintic drugs and thus establishing the adoption of control programs (SATO et al., 2009b).

According to Sato et al. (2009b), in studies on the discrimination of *O. viverrini, C. sinensis, H. pumilio* and *H. taichui*, using nuclear biology techniques aimed at ribosomal DNA extraction and PCR analysis in regions in Thailand, they observed that the difference in size between *O. viverrini* and *C. sinensis* was only around 20 bp (base pairs), using the PCR technique from 4 species of worms. However, according to the authors, it was difficult to use the results to discriminate between the species under study, since only the *H. taichui* amplicon was significantly different in size from the other three species.

3 BIBLIOGRAPHICAL REFERENCES

ANTUNES, S.A.; ALMEIDA DIAS, A. *Phagicola longa* (Trematoda:Heterophyidae) in chilled stored mugilids and their raw consumption in São Paulo, SP.

Food Hygiene, v.8, n.3, 1994.

ANUALPEC -Anuàrio da pecuària brasileira.**FNP consultoria e agroinformativo.** Sâo Paulo - SP, 369 p. 2010.

BARROS. S.B.; AMATO. L.A. Comparative study of lesions observed in *Canis jamiliaris. Fe/is domestica* and *Callithrixjaccnus* experimentally infected with the digenetic *Phagicola longus.* **In: SEMINARIO BRASILEIRO DE** Parasitologia veterinaria, Londrina. 1993.

BENESON, A.S. El control de las enfermedades transmisibles en el hombre.

Washington D.e.: **Organizacion Panamericana de ia Saiud.** (Publicación Cientifica n. 507), 536p. 1987.

BEVILAQUA, C.M.L.; DORCHIES, P. Epidemiological Sunrey of bovine onchocercosis in Southeastem France. **Revista Brasiieira de Parasitoiogia Veterinària,** 145 -150, 1999a.

BEVILAQUA, C.M.L.; P. DORCHIES. Présence d'*Onchocerca lienalis* chez lês bovines en France. **Revue Médicine Vétérinaire,** 1999b.

BEYTUT, E.; ACKA, A.; BAIN, O. Teat onchocercosis in cows with reference to prevalence, species involved and pathology. *Research Veterinary Science*, 78:45-51, 2005.

BIANCHIN, I. **Some factors that interfere with the control of bovine helminths**. In: SEMINARIO NACIONAL SOBRE PARASITOSES DOS BOVINOS, I., 1979, Campo Grande. Proceedings... Campo Grande : EMBRAPA- CNPGC/ CNPq/ PRONAPESA, p.99-111. 1979.

BIONDI, G. F.; HENRIQUE, C. H.; OLIVEIRA, A. C.; CASTRO, A. P. Avaliaçâo CABARET, J.; GEERTS, S.; MADELINE, M.; BALLAN-DONNE, C.; BARBIER, D. The use of urban sewage sludge on pastures: the cysticercosis threat. **Veterinary Research.** v. 33, n. 5, p. 575-597, 2002.

CARPIO, A. Neurocysticercosis: an update. **Lancet Infectious Diseases**, v. 2, 2002.

CASTRO, J.M. **Extraction of *Pllagicola* metacercariae cysts Faust, 1920 (Trematoda: Heterophydae) from *MugiL* Linnaeus, 1758 (Pisces: Mugilidae) mullet tissues using enzymatic digestion and homogenization techniques.** São Paulo. 1994.

CDC/ATLANTA/USA. CENTERS FOR DISEASE CONTROL AND PREVENTION. *Identification and Diagnosis of Parasites of Public Health Concern.* In: **http://www.dpd.cdc.gov/dpdx, 2003**. Accessed on 10/05/2010.

CHIEFFI, P.P.; LEITE. O.H.; DIAS, R.M.D.S.; TORRES, D.M.A.V; MA. Human pamsitism by *Phagicola* sp. (Tremaloda, Heterophyidae) in Cananéia. Sao Paulo Slate, Brazil. **Revista do**

Instituto de Medicina Tropical de Sao Paulo. v.32, p.285. 1990.

CONROY, A. Investigaciones sobre la fagicolosis em lisas (Mugilidae) de águas americanas. I. Taxonomic studies of Phagicola spp. (Trematoda: Heterophyidae) in South American mugilids, *Rev. Iber. Parasitol.* **46**, pp. 3946, 1986.

DIAS, E.R.A.; WOICIECHOVSKJ, E. Occurrence of *Pagicola longa* (Trematoda: Heterophyidae) in mllgilids and man, in Registro and Cananéia, SP.

Food Hygiene. v.8, n.31, pA3-6, 1994.

DOHNAL, J.; BLINN, J.; WAHL, G.; SCHULTZ-KEY, H. Distribution of microfilariae of *Onchocerca lienalis* and *Onchocerca gutturosa* in the skin of cattle in Germany and their development in *Simulium ornatum and Culicoides nubeculosus* following artificial infestation. **Veterinary Parasitology**, 36:325-332, 1990.

DORNY, P.; PRAET, N. *Taenia saginata* in Europe. **Veterinary Parasitology**. v. 149, p. 22-24, 2007.

DUNG, D.T.; WAIKAGUL, J.; DALSGAARD, A.; CHAI, J. Y. "Fishborne zoonotic intestinal trematodes, Vietnam". Emerg Infect Diseasis. Available at http://www.cdc.gov/EID/content/13121828.htm / 2007.

EIRAS, J.C. Elementos de ictioparasitologia. Porto: **Eng. António de Almeida Foundation,** 1994b.

FAUST, E.; BEAVER, P.e.; JUNG, R.C. Agentes e vectores animais de doenças humanas. Porto: **Calousle Gulbenkian Foundation,** 1987.

FLISSER, A.; SARTI, E.; LIGHTOWLERS, M.; SCHANTZ, P. Neurocysticercosis: regional status, epidemiology, impact and control measures in the Americas. **Acta Tropica.** v. 87, n.1, p. 43-51, 2005.

FORTES, E. **Parasitologia veterinària.** 4ª ed. Sao Paulo: icone, 2004.

FUKUDA, R. T.; SANTOS, I. F.; ANDRADE, C. R. Comparative study of the diaphragm inspection technique for the diagnosis of bovine cysticercosis. **Food Hygiene.** v.12, n° 55, p.51-62, 1998.

GEMMELL, M., MATYAS, Z., PAWLOWSKI, Z. et al. (Ed.). **Guidelines for surveillance prevention and control of taeniasis/ cysticercosis.** Geneva:

GUDERIAN, R.H.; ANSELMI, M.; CHICO, H. M.; COOPER, P. J. Onchocerciasis in Ecuador: dermal depigmentation, leopard skin and comparison with treponemal infection. **Parasitologia al dia** v.22 n.1-2 Santiago, 1992.

KASSAI, T. **Veterinary helminthology.** Oxford: Butterworth-Heinemann, 1999.

MARK, L. E. Studies on the Onchocerca found in cattle in the United States. In: Systematics of O.

gutturosa and O. lienalis with a description of O. stilese.

Journal of Parasitology. 65 (3), 379-388, 1979.

MINOZZO, J.; GUSSO, R.L.; CASTRO, E.C.; LAGO, O.; THOMAZ-SOCCOL, V. Experimental bovine infection with Taenia saginata eggs: recovery rate and cysticerci localization. **Brazilian Archives of Biology and Technology,** v. 45, n. 4, p. 451-455, 2002.

MONTEIRO, L. L.; PINTO, P. S. A.; SALCEDO, J. H. P.; ARAÙJO, J.V.;SANTOS, W. L. M. *Taenia solium* larval antigens in ELISA for the diagnosis of bovine cysticercosis. **Arquivo Brasileiro de Medicina Veterinària e Zootecnia.** v.59, n.1, p.21-25, 2007.

OGBOGU, V.C.; BABLIS, J.M.; AJANUSI, O.J. Prevalence of microfilariae in cattle at slaughter in Zaria, Nigeria. **Veterinary Parasitology** 36, 171-175, 1990.

OKUMURA, M.P.M.; PÉREZ, A.C.; FILHO, A. E. Main parasitic zoonoses transmitted by fish - a review. **CRMV-SP Continuing Education Magazine.** *CRMV-SP,* Sao Paulo, volume 2, 1999.

PANAMERICAN HEALTH ORGANIZATION. **Epidemiology and control of teniasis/cysticercosis in Latin America.** Washington: PAHO/WHO, 297p.

1994.

PEREZ, K. A report on the experimental infection of a smooth-headed capuchin monkey *(Ceblls apella)* with metacercarie of *Phagicola longa* obtained from silver mullet *(Mugil curema)* viscera. **Rivista Italiana Piscicultura.** 1985.

PAIVA, F.; HERMANO, J.H.; CARMO, R.G.; LIMA, M.; RIBEIRO, H.S. Oncocerciase bovina no Estado de Mato Grosso do Sul. **Pesquisa Veterinària Brasileira**, v. 4 p. 33 - 37, 1984.

PIERRE, P.P. Emerging diseases, zoonoses and vaccines to control them. **Publications Department, World Organization for Animal Health (OIE)**, 2009.

REY, L. *Onchocerca volvulus* and onchocerciasis. Other filariases. In: . _

Parasitogy: parasites and parasitic diseases of man in the western tropics. 4. ed. Rio de Janeiro: Guanabara Koogan, Chap. 51. pp. 661-675, 2008.

REZENDE, R. B. C.; FERNANDEZ, A. T.; COSTA, F.; SILVA, T. J. P. SANTIN-DURAN, M.; ALUNDA, J.M.; SAN MIGUEL, J.M.; HOBERG, E.P. Elaeophorosis in red deer from Spain. *Journal Wildl Disease*, 15:273-280, 1979.

SANTOS, A. S. O.; LEMOS, L. S.; MATOS, W. R.; MOREIRA, L.; CARVALHO, E. C. Q. Generalized canine *cysticercosis (Cysticercus cellulosae)*. **Ciência Animal Brasileira**, v. 5, n. 4, p. 195-198, 2004.

SANTOS, A.L. Prevention and contrai of food borne trematodes in cultured fish. **INFO FISH International.** n.2, p.57-62, 1995.

SARAIVA, M.E.V. **Estudio de diferentes métodos de conservación sobre la sobrevivencia de metacercarias de *Phagicola longa* Caracas**. Venezuela, 1991.

SATO, M. O.; NAKAO, M.; SAKO, Y.; NAKAYA,K.; QIU, D.; MAMUTI, W; CRAIG, P. S.; ITO, A. DNA differential diagnosis of taenisis and cysticercosis by multiplex PCR. **Journal of Clinical Microbiology**, v. 42, n. 2, p. 548-553, 2004. SATO, M.; THAENKHAM, U.; DEKUMYOY, P.; WAIKAGUL, J. Discrimination of *O. viverrini, C. sinensis, H. pumilio* and *H. taichui* using nuclear DNA-based PCR targeting ribosomal DNA ITS regions. **Acta Tropica,** v.109, p.81-83, 2009a.

SATO, M; SANGUANKIAT, S.; PUBAMPEN S.; KUSOLSUK, T.; MAIPANICH, W.; WAIKAGUL, J. **Egg Laying Capacity of** *Haplorchis taichui* **(Digenea: Heterophyidae) in Humans.** Department of Helminthology, Faculty of Tropical Medicine, Mahidol University, 420/6 Rachawithi Road, Rachathewee, Bangkok 10400, Thailand. Korean J Parasitol. September; 47(3): 315-318, 2009b.

SCHANTZ, P.M.; CRUZ, M.; SARTI, E.; PAWLOWSKI, S. Z. The potential eradicability of teniasis and cysticercosis. **Boletin de la Oficina Sanitaria Panamericana**, v.116, n.5, p.465-469, 1994.

SILVA, A. V. M. Teniasis and Cysticercosis. In: NEVES, D. P. **Human Parasitology**. 8. ed. Sao Paulo: Livraria Atheneu, 462p. 2005.

SINGH, B. Molecular methods for diagnosis and epidemiological studies of parasitic infections. **International Journal for Parasitology**, v. 27, n. 10, p.11351145, 1997.

SOLISMAA, M.; LAAKSONEN, S.; NYLUND, M.; PITKÄNEN, E.; AIRAKORPI, R.; OKSANEN, A. Filarioid nematodes in cattle, sheep and horses in Finland. Acta Veterinaria Scandinavica. http://www.actavetscand.com/content/50/1/20 accessed on 24/08/2009 09:05 20 - 50, 2008.

SOMERS, R.; DORNY, P.; NGUYEN, V. K.; DANG, T. C. T.; GODEERIS, B.; CRAIG, P. S.; VERCRUYSSE, J. *Taenia solium* taeniasis and cysticercosis in three communities in north Vietnam. **Tropical Medicine and International Health**, v. 2, n. 1, p. 65-72, 2006.

SOUZA, V. K.; PESSOA-SILVA, M. C.; KOWALCZUK, M. Anatomical regions of higher occurrence of *Cysticercus bovis* in cattle submitted to federal inspection in a slaughterhouse-frigorifico in the municipality of Sao José dos Pinhais, Paranà, from July to December 2000. **Revista Brasileira de Parasitologia Veterinària.** v.16, n.2, p.92-96, 2007.

SOUZA,R.M.; ANTUNES,C.F.; GUATIMOSIM, C. The importance of the federal inspection service in food health surveillance - Bovine cysticercosis.

Food Hygiene. v.11 n° 48, 1978.

THATCHER, V.E.; NETO, J.B. Diagnosis, prevention and treatment of neotropical freshwater fish diseases. **Revista Brasileira de Medicina Veterinària.** v.16 n.3, 1994.

TRESS, A.J.; GRAHAM, S.P.; S.; RENZ, A.; TANYA, V. *Onchocerca ochengi* infections in cattle as a model for human onchocerciasis: recent developments. **Parasitology today** 120, 133-142, 2000.

TRESS, A.J.; WAHL, G; KLAGER, S.; RENZ, A. Age-related differences in parasitosis may indicate acquired immunity against microfilariae in cattle naturally infected with *Onchocerca ochengi*. **Parasitology today** 104, 247-252, 1992.

UNGAR, M.L.; GERMANO, P.M.L. Prevalence of bovine cysticercosis in the state of São Paulo (Brazil). **Revista Saùde Pùblica**, v.26 n°. 3, p.167-172, 1992.

URQUHART, G.M.; ARMOUR, J.; DUNCAN, J.L.; DUNN, A.M.; JENNINGS, F.W. **Parasitologia veterinària** 2 ed. p.89 Rio de Janeiro: Guanabara Koogan, 2008.

WILDENBURG, G.; PLENGE-BONIG, A.; RENZ, A.; FISCHER, P.; BUTTNER, D. W. Distribution of mast cells and their correlation with inflammatory cells around *Onchocerca gutturosa, O. tarsicola, O. ochengi* and *O. flexuosa*. **Parasitology Research** 83, 109-120, 1997.

WORLD HEALTH ORGANIZATION - **WHO**. Control of neurocysticercosis. Fifty-Fifth World Health Assembly A 55/23 provisional. in: ORGANIZATION OF THE UNITED NATIONS, **2002**. Available at: www.who.int/gb/ebwha/pdf _files /WHA55 /ea5523.pdf. Accessed: Jan. 2010

CHAPTER I

Occurrence of *Onchocerca* spp. in beef cattle in the northern region of the state of Tocantins.

SUMMARY

Some species of *Onchocerca spp.* are agents of important zoonoses. This study verified the occurrence of onchocerciasis in beef cattle raised extensively in the northern region of Brazil, specifically in the northern state of Tocantins. Material was analyzed from 104 cattle slaughtered and inspected under the Federal Inspection Service of Frigorifico Boi Forte (SIF 723), located in Araguaina - TO, from the municipalities of Bernardo Sayâo, Araguanâ, Pau D'arco, Arapoema, Carmolândia, Muricilândia and Santa Fé do Araguaia, of different breeds and coats, mostly male and aged over 36 months. The samples collected for analysis were from cervical ligaments, navels and blood. All the samples analyzed were negative, both for adult parasites in the cervical ligaments and for microfilariae in the blood and navel samples. No lesions or nodules were found in the cervical ligaments of the animals studied, nor any visible changes during the course of this work. Therefore, onchocerciasis was not found in the cattle analyzed in this region.

Key words: Helminths, microfilariae, cervical ligament, connective tissue, filariasis

1 INTRODUCTION

Nematodes are called cylindrical worms because of their appearance in cross-section. They are based on ten superfamilies in which nematodes of veterinary importance occur, including the Filarioidea, whose main representatives are the following nematodes: *Dirofilaria, Onchocerca, Parafilaria.* These nematodes typically have slender, long bodies, an indirect evolutionary cycle and are infected by the L3 (infective larva) of insects (URQUHART, 2008).

The effects of nematodes on cattle depend on the species and the degree of infection, which in turn depends on various factors, such as: climatic conditions, soil, vegetation, type of farm, breed, age of the animal and type of pasture. However, in extensive beef cattle breeding in Central Brazil, worm infestation is a contributing factor to the animals' low growth rate (BIANCHIN, 1979).

Beef cattle farming in the state of Tocantins is of great importance in Brazilian agribusiness as it is one of the main sources of income in the country's northern region, with the presence of small, medium and large cattle farmers (ANUALPEC, 2006). In this context, Tocantins is one of the main beef supply centers for both the domestic and foreign markets.

According to ANUALPEC (2006), the state of Tocantins produced more than 220,000 tons of carcass equivalent. However, onchocerciasis is a disease caused by helminths of the genus *Onchocerca* spp. that can be present in cattle raised extensively in northern Brazil, specifically in the northern state of Tocantins.

The occurrence of a variety of filarid species in cattle is widely distributed geographically. Filarioid nematodes are known to occur in domestic animals all over the world. The most abundant and economically important species found in cattle are *Onchocerca gibsoni, O. gutturosa, O. armillata, O. lienalis, O. ochengi, O. bovicola, Parafilaria spp.* and *Stephanofilaria spp.* Generally, the species of *Onchocerca* spp, are medium-sized filarids that normally inhabit the subcutaneous tissues, ligaments and aponeuroses of large mammals, producing microfilariae on the skin and in the bloodstream (OGBOGU et al., 1990).

The definitive hosts of most species of these helminths are generally well adapted and tolerate the presence of the parasites in their bodies. For example, *Onchocerca* spp. in cattle in Africa generally show low pathogenicity. Normally, the damage caused by filarid worms is an inflammatory reaction around dead helminths or microfilariae. These, in turn, present in the subcutaneous tissue, calcify and become surrounded by dense fibrous tissue, causing little damage (WAHL et al., 1994).

Human onchocerciasis, on the other hand, is caused by a parasitic worm that can lead to blindness. The adult worms are found coiled inside fibrous, subcutaneous tumors called onchocerciasis nodules. When they reproduce, the worms produce a large quantity of microfilariae, which migrate into the subcutaneous tissue and are then ingested by hematophagous insects (simuliids). The typical nodules can be found anywhere on the body, but are more frequent near the joints and on the head (REY, 2008).

Simuliids, commonly known as borrachudos or piùns, belong to the group Diptera, family Simuliidae. Known in the past for the aggressiveness of their adult females, they are now known to be vectors of viruses, protozoa and worms, causing serious health problems for humans and animals (MAIA-HERZOG, 1999).

The aim of this study was to assess the occurrence of onchocerciasis in beef cattle slaughtered in the northern region of the state of Tocantins, a zoonosis that is still little known in terms of its occurrence and routes of transmission, as well as to check for the presence of this parasite in cattle from surrounding municipalities slaughtered at the Boi Forte meatpacking plant in Araguaina - TO, as there has been no study of this parasitic nematode in the region.

2 MATERIAL AND METHODS

2.1 Experiment site and sample collection

The experiment was conducted at the Parasitology Laboratory of the School of Veterinary Medicine and Zootechnics of the Federal University of Tocantins (UFT) and on the premises of the Boi Forte meatpacking plant, located in Araguaina - TO, from September 2009 to January 2010.

Materials were collected weekly from cattle slaughtered and inspected by the Federal Inspection Service of Frigorifico Boi Forte (SIF - 723), from the municipalities of Bernardo Sayâo, Araguanâ, Pau D'arco, Arapoema, Carmolândia, Muricilândia and Santa Fé do Araguaia, of different breeds and coats, mostly male cattle aged over 36 months (Table 1). The samples collected for analysis were from cervical ligaments (for research into adult parasites), navels and blood (for research into microfilariae), totaling 104 animals.

The cervical ligament and umbilicus samples were packed and identified separately in plastic bags, and the umbilicus samples were preserved in 10% formaldehyde for further processing. The blood samples were collected directly from the jugular vein, where the animals were bled, with anticoagulant in test tubes (EDTA - 1 mL / tube) and stored under refrigeration at 4° C.

For all collections, the times at which the samples were to be taken were stipulated, so that they occurred randomly according to the batch that was being slaughtered at the time of collection.

During the research, the presence of *Onchocerca* spp. in cattle slaughtered at this establishment was evaluated, observing the following criteria: sex, breed, age, origin of the animals slaughtered and the verification of lesions caused by the parasite.

The presence of *Onchocerca* spp. was investigated in the samples and the results were related to the sex, breed, age, coat and origin of the animals, as can be seen in Table 1.

Table 1 - List of cervical ligament, navel and blood samples collected at the Boi Forte slaughterhouse (SIF 723) during the period from 18/09/2009 to 20/01/2010.

PROCEDURE	N° OF ANIMALS	RACE	COAT	SEX	AGE	NOTE
Faz. Jatoba mun. Bernardo Sayâo Prop. Cian Cia Ind. Alimentos	10	Nelore	White	F	>36 M	18/09/2009
Faz. Caxingui Mun. Muricilândia Prop. Rubens S. Souza C. Jûnior	10	Nelore	White	M	>36M	28/09/2009

Faz. Santa Rita Mun. Pau D'arco Prop. Luis A. C. Soares	10	½ Angus X Nelore	Black	M	>36 M	16/11/2009
Faz. Eldorado Municipality of Arapoema Prop. Alexandre Jûlio de Albuquerque Maranhâo	15	Nelore	White	M	>36 M	23/11/2009
Faz. Maria Rosa Santa Fé Prop. Sèrgio A. C. Castro	15	Nelore	White	M	>36 M	13/01/2010
Faz. Vista Alegre Municipality of Araguanâ Prop. Francisco Tude M. Neto	20	Nelore	White	M	>36 M	14/01/2010
Flôr da Mata Farm Carmolândia Prop. Maria de Lourdes N. Adriano	24	½ Red Angus X Nelore	Gust	M	>36 M	20/01/2010
TOTAL ANIMALS COLLECTED = 104						

It is worth noting that all the properties mentioned above carry out strategic control of helminths in cattle with the use of ivermectin, as recommended by Bianchin (1979) for Central Brazil.

2.2 Laboratory tests

For the analysis of the cervical ligaments (figures 3 to 5), the technique described by Ottley & Moorhouse (1979) was followed. The analysis of blood (figure 6) followed the Knott's technique, modified to check for microfilariae.

A microscopic analysis of the navels collected for microfilariae was also carried out by making histological slides and staining them with H.E. (Hematoxylin-Eosin).

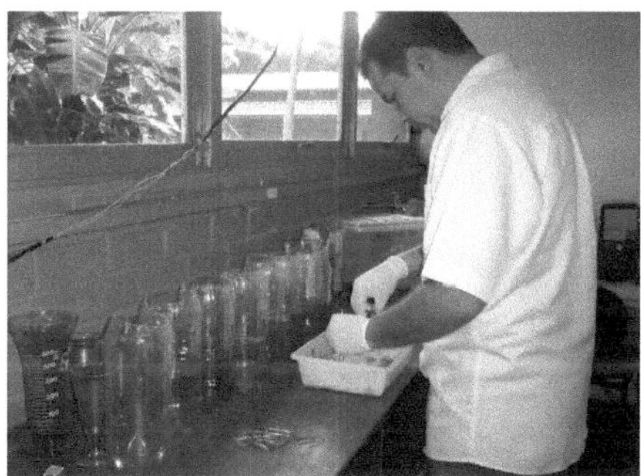

Figure 1 - Preparation of materials for digestion in pepsin.

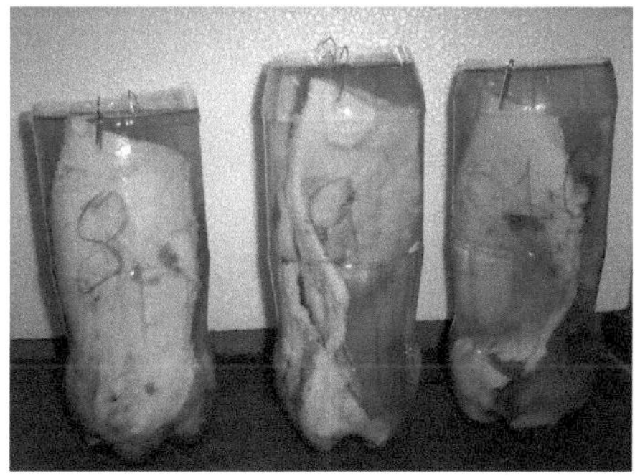

Figure 2 - Cervical ligament processing of cattle for digestion.

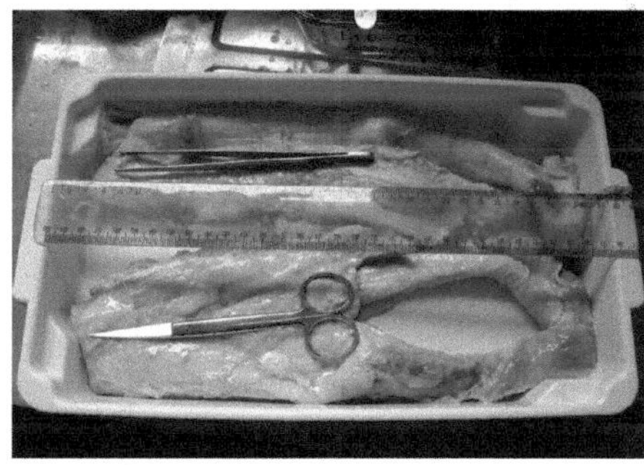

Figure 3 - Bovine cervical ligament

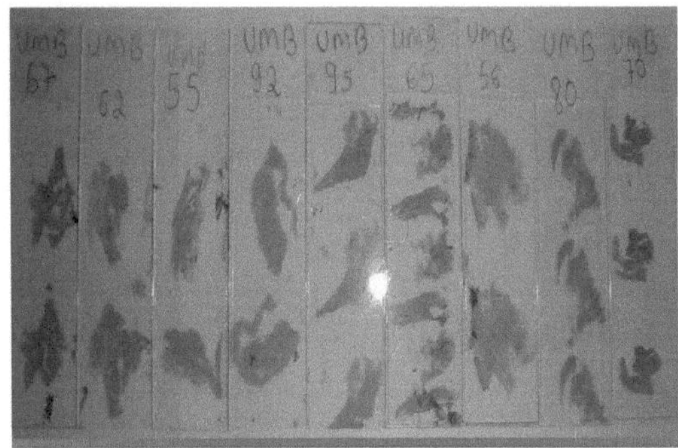

Figure 4 - Histological slides of navels (stain: H.E.)

3   RESULTS AND DISCUSSION

All the samples analyzed were negative (100%), both for adult parasites (in the cervical ligaments) and for microfilariae (in the blood and navels). No lesions or nodules were found in the cervical ligaments of the animals surveyed, nor any visible changes during the course of this work.

The absence of adult parasites and microfilariae of *Onchocerca* spp. in cattle slaughtered in the northern region of the state of Tocantins, in all the samples from the 104 animals, indicates that this disease may not occur in the region mentioned, given that the samples were collected randomly, although the presence of the mosquito vector (*Simulium* spp.) in rural properties in the region has been verified.

The results found here differ from those observed by other authors, especially Paiva et al (1984), in a study carried out in the state of Mato Grosso do Sul, where the prevalence of *Onchocerca* spp. in the cervical ligaments of cattle slaughtered in slaughterhouses was 100%. Only one species was found in this study, *Onchocerca gutturosa.* The author also comments that the animals parasitized by these nematodes, even at a high level of infection, did not show any obvious clinical manifestations.

In Finland, *Onchocerca* spp. microfilariae were found in skin samples from cattle slaughtered in slaughterhouses, with a high prevalence of 37% (SOLISMAA et al., 2008).

However, in Europe, infections in cattle by *Onchocerca* spp. are very abundant, for example, in Germany the prevalence of microfilariae in a study of slaughtered cattle was 40.4%. The study was carried out on animals aged between 14 and 143 months. In all of them, the presence of microfilariae and macroscopic lesions were observed in various tissues with a greenish-gray color and the presence of edema, as well as small nodules in most of the lesions (SOLISMAA et al., 2008).

According to Wahl et al. (1994), in studies of skin biopsies from the umbilical region of 204 cattle in northern Cameroon, the presence of *Onchocerca gutturosa, O. ochengi* and *O. dukei* microfilariae was observed in 85%, 51% and 8% of the samples collected, respectively. In another study, in the savannahs of Sudan, the same authors found the same species of microfilariae, in higher proportions than those described above, 92%, 83% and 47%, respectively.

4   CONCLUSION

The presence of adult parasites and microfilariae of *Onchocerca* spp. in cattle slaughtered in the northern region of the state of Tocantins was not detected in any of the 104 animals sampled in this study. This shows us that this disease may not occur in the region mentioned, given that the samples were collected randomly. Even so, it is worth noting that the mosquito vector (*Simulium* spp.) has been found on rural properties in the region.

5   BIBLIOGRAPHICAL REFERENCES

ANUALPEC - Brazilian livestock yearbook. **FNP consultoria e agroinformativo.** Sâo Paulo - SP, 369 p. 2006.

BIANCHIN, I. **Some factors that interfere with the control of helminths in cattle.** In: SEMINARIO NACIONAL SOBRE PARASITOSES DOS BOVINOS, I., 1979, Campo Grande. Proceedings... Campo Grande: EMBRAPA-CNPGC/CNPq/PRONAPESA, p.99-111. 1979.

MAIA-HERZOG, M. Human onchocerciasis in Brazil and its spread. PhD thesis in parasitic biology. Rio de Janeiro, National School of Public Health, **Oswaldo Cruz Institute, Fiocruz.** 1999.

OGBOGU, V.C.; BABLIS, J.M.; AJANUSI, O.J. Prevalence of microfilariae in cattle at slaughter in Zaria, Nigeria. **Veterinary Parasitology** 36, 171-175, 1990.

OTTLEY, M. L.; MOORHOUSE, D. E. *Onchocerca* (Nematoda: Filarioidea) from Queensland cattle; redescription of *Onchocerca gibsoni* (Cleland and Johnston) and *O. lienalis.* Zoologister anzeiger 203 (5/6): 369-377, 1979.

PAIVA, F.; HERMANO, J.H.; CARMO, R.G.; LIMA, M.; RIBEIRO, H.S. Oncocerciase bovina no Estado de Mato Grosso do Sul. **Pesquisa Veterinària Brasileira**, v. 4 p. 33 - 37, 1984.

REY, L. *Onchocerca volvulus* and onchocerciasis. Other filariases. In: . __

Parasitogy: parasites and parasitic diseases of man in the western tropics. 4. ed. Rio de Janeiro: Guanabara Koogan, Chap. 51. pp. 661-675, 2008.

SOLISMAA, M.; LAAKSONEN, S.; NYLUND, M.; PITKANEN, E.; AIRAKORPI, R.;

OKSANEN, A. Filarioid nematodes in cattle, sheep and horses in Finland. *Acta Veterinaria Scandinavica.* http://www.actavetscand.com/content/50/1/20 accessed on 24/08/2009 09:05, 2008.

URQUHART, G.M.; ARMOUR, J.; DUNCAN, J.L.; DUNN, A.M.; JENNINGS, F.W.

Parasitologia veterinària 2 ed. p.89 Rio de Janeiro: Guanabara Koogan, 2008.

WAHL, G.; ACHU-KWI, M.D.; MBAH, D.; DAWA, O.; RENZ, A. Bovine onchocercosis in north Cameroon. **Veterinary Parasitology.** v.52, p. 297-311, 1994.

CHAPTER II

Search for Heterophyidae metacercariae in Amazonian fish
(*Leporinus fasciatus*).

SUMMARY

The occurrence of Heterophiidae metacercariae in Amazonian fish (*Leporinus fasciatus*) was verified, as parasitic zoonoses transmitted by fish are drawing increasing attention from researchers and health authorities around the world, due to the occurrence of public health problems in the population, which becomes infected through the consumption of raw or insufficiently cooked fish. Zoonoses transmissible by fish include anisakiasis, eustrongylidiasis, capillariasis, phagicolosis, clonorchiasis and diphyllobothriasis, among others. Metacercariae were recovered from 65 fish specimens (piau-flamengo), which were then inoculated into hamsters and ducks to recover the adult parasite. The main measure to prevent infection by these parasites is to abstain from eating raw or undercooked fish. There is still a need to educate and raise awareness among the population, alerting them to the potential dangers of eating raw fish, as well as developing reliable techniques for inspecting and processing fish infected with parasites, in order to offer greater safety to the population. These parasites have a life cycle in which humans can be the definitive host, where infection is usually asymptomatic. The results obtained in this study showed that most of the animals evaluated were positive for the presence of the parasite. However, with this research, metacercariae that are potential pathogens for public health were detected in fish for human consumption, but it was not possible to confirm the species of trematode and further studies on these parasites are needed.

Keywords: *Heterophyidae*, zoonosis, metacercaria and fish.

1   INTRODUCTION

The *Heterophyidae* family described in Brazil is represented by 11 species, distributed in six genera. They are small trematodes whose definitive hosts are birds and mammals, including man and, occasionally, reptiles (THATCHER and NETO, 1994).

Infection in humans is generally asymptomatic in the early stages, and the impact on health is directly proportional to the parasite load. On the other hand, chronic infections with these intestinal trematodes cause bile retention in the intra- and extra-biliary tract, as well as dilatation, inflammation of the ducts, suppurative cholangitis, abscesses and fibrosis. Malignant transformation of the duct epithelium (cholangiocarcinoma) has also been reported as a result of the final complications of parasitism (OLIVEIRA, et al., 2007).

In this way, heterophiids are of considerable importance in public health, especially when it comes to transporting live fish, as is the case with ornamental fish. They can transport disease-causing agents from endemic areas to disease-free areas, as well as introducing new pathogens with zoonotic potential to a new region (THATCHER and NETO, 1994).

According to Anualpec (2010), fish production in the state of Tocantins in 2007 was 1,667 tons from extractive fishing and 4,458 tons from farmed fish.

In fish, metacercariae are usually attached to the skin or gills, where they remain alive for months. The metacercariae are unicellular, surrounded by two walls. The inner wall is thin and transparent, covering the entire structure, while the outer wall is made of protein, covering the dorsal and lateral surfaces (OLIVEIRA, et al., 2007).

Parasitic zoonoses transmitted by fish are increasingly attracting the attention of researchers and health authorities around the world, due to the occurrence of public health problems in the population, which becomes infected through the consumption of raw or insufficiently cooked fish (OKUMURA et al).

Although zoonoses transmitted by trematodes through the consumption of fish cause liver diseases, which have been well documented in Vietnam, those that affect the intestine have an under-described occurrence. Recent research into the presence of metacercariae of human intestinal trematode parasites in fish caught and farmed in Vietnam has shown that there is a potential risk for communities that consume raw fish (SATO et al., 2009a).

It should be noted that there are studies using molecular methods for the direct diagnosis of metacercariae, making it possible to ascertain the species of parasites that occur in the region with greater specificity. The aim of this study was to investigate the presence of parasites that cause zoonoses in Amazonian fish and to recover adult and immature trematodes and metacercariae from Amazonian fish heterophiids.

2 MATERIAL AND METHODS

2.1 Experiment site

The experiment was conducted on the premises of the Parasitology Laboratory of the School of Veterinary Medicine and Zootechnics (EMVZ) of the Federal University of Tocantins (UFT), from January to July 2010.

2.2 Obtaining fish and collecting metacercariae

The fish of the species *Leporinus fasciatus* (Flemish piau) were purchased at the Araguaina - TO municipal market between March and July 2010, totaling 65 specimens. The fish collected had already been sacrificed and their viscera discarded. They were stored at 4°C until analysis in the Parasitology laboratory.

2.3 Metacercaria recovery

Each fish was carefully examined in order to find metacercariae in the muscles and fins, using the pepsin digestion technique. To do this, the tissue samples (muscles, skin, scales and bones) were digested in pepsin (1% pepsin solution in distilled water with HCl, pH 2) and incubated for 3-4 hours in an oven at 37°C.

After digestion, the samples were sieved and the filtrate was washed in 0.85% saline and examined under a stereoscopic microscope.

To test for parasites in fish fins, they were digested and washed, as it was found that metacercariae are usually embedded in the fin rays.

The recovered metacercariae were stored in 2 mL micro tubes (Eppendorf) with 0.85% saline solution for later inoculation in hamsters and ducks, with the aim of recovering the adult forms of the parasite.

2.4 Experimental inoculation of metacercariae in hamsters

For the experimental infections, two hamsters (*Mesocricetus auratus*) were used and given 51 metacercariae orally. A disposable 3 mL syringe attached to a probe was used for administration. The first animal was infected on 23/03/2010 and the second on 29/03/2010. After infection, the animals were immunosuppressed with 0.1 ml of methylprednizolone (40 mg/ml) for 3 consecutive days.

Throughout the experimental period, the animals were kept in experimental cages with water and feed *ad libitum* and every two days the "bedding" in the boxes was changed.

Fecal examinations of these animals were carried out daily during the 5 days of the experiment, using the Hoffmann technique (sedimentation). This examination was carried out in order to check for the presence of possible trematode eggs (Heterophiideos) in the infected animals.

On the 5th day after each inoculation, euthanasia was carried out using carbon dioxide (CO_2). The animals were analyzed for the recovery of the adult form of trematodes (Heterophiidae). The necropsy of each animal was carried out in the parasitology laboratory and the following organs were analyzed: stomach, intestines, heart, lungs, kidneys and liver.

2.5 Experimental inoculation of metacercariae in ducks

Research into trematode parasites was carried out using ducks (*Anas platyrhynchos*) as an experimental model, with the aim of recovering adult parasites. To this end, two three-day-old ducks, acquired from the Gota de Mel property in the rural area of Araguaina - TO, were subjected to fecal examination using the Willis and Hoffmann techniques before being infected.

The infection procedure was the same as that used with hamsters (except for the immunosuppressant applications). The first animal was inoculated on 23/06/2010 and 5 days after infection the same euthanasia technique was used as in item 3.4. The second animal was infected on 02/07/2010 and euthanized 3 days after the date of infection.

After euthanasia, the adult form of trematodes was recovered, which was carried out as described in section 3.4. During the necropsy of these animals, the following organs were analyzed: aglandular (gizzard) and glandular stomach, intestines, heart and liver.

2.6 Measuring the size of recovered metacercariae

A sample was taken of the size of the metacercariae recovered in order to find out their real size. Table 1 describes the measurements taken.

Table 1 - Sizing of metacercariae - MTC (smallest diameter, largest diameter and size) recovered from Amazonian fish of the species *Leporinus fasciatus* (piau-flamengo) in the municipality of Araguaina - TO, 2010.

TCM	Smallest diameter (mm)	Size (µm)	Largest diameter (mm)	Size (µm)
1	2,0	197,8	2,1	207,69
2	1,8	178,02	1,9	187,91
3	1,8	178,02	1,9	187,91
4	1,9	187,91	2,0	197,8
5	1,8	178,02	1,9	187,91
6	2,2	217,58	2,2	217,58
7	1,9	187,91	2,0	197,8
8	1,9	187,91	1,9	187,91
9	1,8	178,02	1,9	187,91
10	1,9	187,91	2,1	207,69
11	1,8	178,02	1,9	187,91

12	1,9	187,91	2,0	197,8
13	2,2	217,58	2,2	217,58
14	1,7	168,13	1,8	178,02
15	1,9	187,91	1,9	187,91
16	1,8	178,02	2,0	197,8
17	1,9	187,91	2,0	197,8
18	2,0	197,8	2,1	207,69
19	2,2	217,58	2,2	217,58
20	1,7	168,13	1,8	178,02
Average	1.9 cm	188.40 µm	1.99 cm	196.81µm

These values were obtained by calculating the Correction Factor, previously calibrated for the microscope used in this analysis. To do this, the metacercariae were measured using a graduated ocular lens and 10x magnification.

3 RESULTS AND DISCUSSION

The results obtained from the metacercariae test on fish from the Araguaia River showed that most of the animals evaluated were positive for the presence of the parasite.

Thus, after enzymatic digestion of the fins, 562 metacercariae were found in the fish observed, with an average of 8.64 metacercariae per fish.

These data suggest that the fish of this species belonging to this region are infected. Table 2 shows the number of metacercariae recovered for each fish analyzed.

The metacercariae obtained in this study were morphologically diagnosed as probable metacercariae of heterophiids.

Considering that this group includes many genera that cause zoonoses, there is a high possibility of infection in humans who consume these fish (SATO et al. 2009b).

No parasites from the *Heterophiidae* family (trematodes) were found in the organs of the hamsters analyzed (stomach, intestines, heart, lungs, kidneys and liver). However, nematode parasites were present in large quantities in the intestines of these animals, which were not identified.

The results of the fecal examinations of the ducks using the Willis and Hoffmann techniques (flotation and sedimentation, respectively) were negative as regards the presence of parasite eggs in the material examined.

No parasites from the *Heterophiidae* family (trematodes) were found in the duck organs analyzed (aglandular (gizzard) and glandular stomachs, intestines, heart and liver); only a few nematodes were present in the samples, but they were not identified.

Several studies have been carried out in order to elucidate the biological cycle of these parasites, using different experimental models. Thus, to evaluate the life cycle of Ascocotyle (Heterophiideo), hamsters were infected with *Phagicola longa,* however the identification of the adult parasite has not been well elucidated (DIAS and WOICIECHOVSKI, 1994; BARROS and AMATO, 1995a; SCHOLZ et al., 2001; DZIKOWSKI et al., 2004).

Table 2 - List of fish (*Leporinus fasciatus* - piau-flamengo) purchased at the Araguaina - TO municipal market and the number of metacercariae (MTC) recovered from their fins between March and July 2010.

Fish	TCM	Fish	TCM
1	1	41	4
2	2	42	7
3	1	43	8
4	6	44	9
5	20	45	11

6	22	46	0
7	71	47	0
8	13	48	0
9	19	49	0
10	7	50	9
11	55	51	8
12	11	52	4
13	7	53	13
14	6	54	10
15	2	55	12
16	3	56	14
17	18	57	11
18	10	58	4
19	19	59	10
20	6	60	15
21	5	61	7
22	2	62	9
23	0	63	8
24	0	64	11
25	6	65	3
26	0	-	-
27	4	-	-
28	12	-	-
29	2	-	-
30	1	-	-
31	7	-	-
32	0	-	-
33	8	-	-
34	6	-	-
35	8	-	-
36	2	-	-
37	11	-	-
38	2	-	-
39	0	-	-
40	0	-	-
Total	375	Tota	187

Grand total of recovered metacercariae = 562

In addition, Hutton (1959) carried out an experimental hamster infection with metacercariae obtained from mullet and suggested that these parasitic forms were related to *P. longa,* but the infected animals did not develop adult *P. longa* parasites.

The wide distribution of *Heleobia australis* molluscs, intermediate hosts of *P. longa,* is believed to be the main reason for the spread of this parasite in the environment. These molluscs are found from Rio de Janeiro to Argentina (DE FRANCESCO and ISLA, 2004).

Thus, the epidemiological consequences can be serious, due to the risk of human infection over a large area (DIAS and WOICIECHOVSKI, 1994). In fact, the impact on public health was confirmed by the high prevalence (100%) of *P. longa* found in mullets examined in urban areas in the state of Rio de Janeiro (VIEIRA, 1991).

Dias and Woiciechovski (1994) also investigated parasitism by *P. longa* in infected mullets in the state of São Paulo. These authors reported that the prevalence of infection increases with the size of the fish as follows: 2.4-4 cm = 0%, 10-13 cm = 60% and > 20 cm = 100%. These data corroborate those obtained by De Francesco, 2004 and Isla, 2004, who reported infection in adult fish from the Rodrigo de Freitas lagoon, between 30-34 cm in length.

Generally, the parasites of the *Mugilidae* family spawn in the open sea and the growth of the juveniles takes place in estuaries and coastal zones, places that provide the necessary conditions for their growth for a large part of their lives. When they mature, they migrate to the sea during the spawning period (VIEIRA, 1991). Therefore, the life cycle of *P. longa* is related to estuaries and coastal lagoons. During the period of migration back to the sea there is an increase in fishing, which can influence the transmission of the parasite to the population (DE FRANCESCO and ISLA, 2004).

Reports indicate that infection by *P. longa* occurs in the muscles of the fish's body (YAMAGUTI, 1975). Considering the large number of oriental restaurants serving raw fish (sashimi, sushi) in large cities such as Rio de Janeiro and São Paulo, the occurrences of infections in humans and in various cities along the Brazilian coast could have a major impact on public health due to infections caused by *P. longa* (VIEIRA, 1991).

It is believed that no adult parasites were found in the experimentally infected animals during this research, because these parasites develop in coastal regions, as has been described by some researchers previously. However, the fish surveyed came from the Araguaia River (freshwater) and there may not have been Phagicola (Trematodes) in these fish, but other types of trematodes that cause zoonoses. Another point worth highlighting is the specificity of the hosts analyzed (hamsters and ducks). It is believed that these did not develop the adult stages of the parasites, due to their lack of specificity to this type of parasite.

Thus, there is a need for further research into these parasites, due to their importance in public health, as metacercariae are the forms of resistance of trematodes, potential agents of gastrointestinal tract diseases in humans.

4 CONCLUSIONS

Fish of the species *Leporinus fasciatus* (piau-flamengo) from this region showed a high prevalence of trematode metacercariae.

5 BIBLIOGRAPHICAL REFERENCES

ANUALPEC - Brazilian livestock yearbook. **FNP consultoria e agroinformativo.** Sâo Paulo - SP, 369 p. 2010.

BARROS, S.B; AMATO, L.A. Aspectos pathológicos observados em hamsters (*Mesocricetus auritus*) infectod cxpcrimcntalmcntc com mctacercàrias *Phagicola longus* (Ransom, 1920) Price, 1932 (Digenea, Heterophyidae), **Revista Brasileira de Parasitologia Veterinària.** *Vol.* **4,** pp. 43-48, 1995a

DE FRANCESCO, C.G.; ISLA, F.I. The life cycle and growth of *Heleobia australis* (d'Orbigny, 1835) and *H. conexa* (Gaillard, 1974) (Gastropoda: Rissooidea) in Mar Chiquita coastal lagoon (Argentina), **Journal Mol. Study.** *v.* **70** pp. 173-178, 2004.

DIAS, E.R.A.; WOICIECHOVSKJ, E. Occurrence of *Pagicola longa* (Trematoda: Heterophyidae) in mllgilids and in man, in Registro and Cananéia, SP. **Food Hygiene.** v.8, n.31, pA3-6, 1994.

DUNG, D.T.; WAIKAGUL, J.; DALSGAARD, A.; CHAI, J. Y. "Fishborne zoonotic intestinal trematodes, Vietnam". Emerg Infect Diseasis. Available at http://www.cdc.gov/EID/content/13121828.htm / 2007.

DZIKOWSKI, R. DZIKOWSKI, M.G. POORE, J.R. Use of rDNA polymorphism for identification of Heterophyidae infecting freshwater fishes. ***Dis. Aquat. Org.*** v. **59** , pp. 35-41, 2004.

HUTTON,R.F. Studies on the trematode parasites encysted in Florida mullets. *State Board Conserv.* **Lab. Spec. Science.** pp. 1-88, 1959.

OLIVEIRA, S.A.; BLAZQUEZ, F.J.H.; ANTUNES, S.A.; MAIA, A.A.M.. Metacercariae of Ascocotyle (Phagicola) longa Ransom, 1920 (Digenea: Heterophyidae), in Mugil platanus, in the Cananéia estuary, SP, Brazil / Ascocotyle (Phagicola) longa Ransom, 1920 (Digenea: Heterophylidae) **Ciência Rural.** v.37, n.4, p.1056-1059, 2007.

OKUMURA, M.P.M.; PÉREZ, A.C.; FILHO, A. E. Main parasitic zoonoses transmitted by fish - a review. **CRMV-SP Continuing Education Magazine.** *CRMV-SP,* Sâo Paulo, volume 2, 1999.

SATO, M; SANGUANKIAT, S.; PUBAMPEN S.; KUSOLSUK, T.; MAIPANICH, W.;

WAIKAGUL, J. **Egg Laying Capacity of** *Haplorchis taichui* **(Digenea: Heterophyidae) in Humans.** Department of Helminthology, Faculty of Tropical Medicine, Mahidol University, 420/6 Rachawithi Road, Rachathewee, Bangkok 10400, Thailand. Korean J Parasitol. September; 47(3): 315-318, 2009a.

SATO, M.; THAENKHAM, U.; DEKUMYOY, P.; WAIKAGUL, J. Discrimination of O. viverrini, C. sinensis, H. pumilio and H. taichui using nuclear DNA-based PCR targeting ribosomal DNA ITS regions. **Acta Tropica,** v.109, p.81-83, 2009b.

SCHOLZ, T.; SCHOLZ, M.L. AGUIRRE-MACEDO, G. Trematodes of the family Heterophyidae

(Digenea) in Mexico: a review of species and new host and geographical records, *Journal National History* v. **35** pp. 1733-1772, 2001.

THATCHER, V.E.; NETO, J.B. Diagnosis, prevention and treatment of neotropical freshwater fish diseases. Revista Brasileira de Medicina Veterinària, v.16 n.3, 1994.

VIEIRA, J. *Juveniles mullets* (Pisces: Mugilidae) in the estuary of Lagoa dos Patos, RS, *Brazil.* pp. 409-418. 1991.

YAMAGUTI, S. Review of Life Histories of Digenetic Trematodes of Vertebrates, Keigaku Publ. Co., Tokyo, Japan. 590p. 1975.

6 ANNEXES

RANCH 1

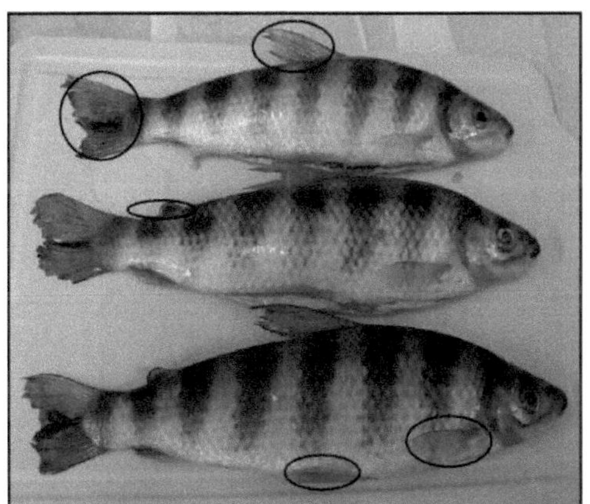

Figure 1 - Fish of the species *Leporinus fasciatus* (Flemish Piau)

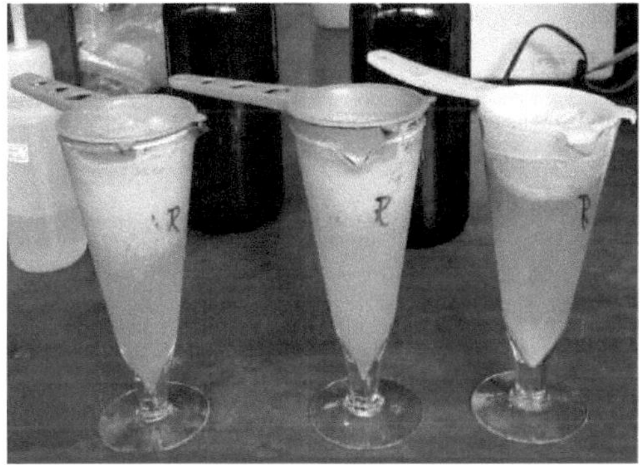

Figure 2 - Digestion of muscles, skin, scales and bones in 1% pepsin to recover metacercariae.

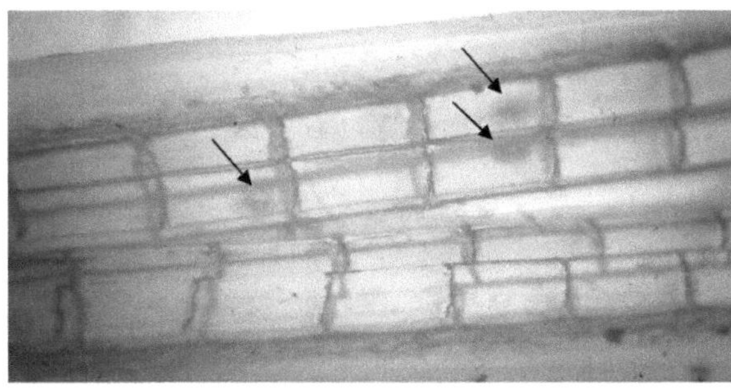

Figure 3 - Metacercariae embedded in the fin rays.

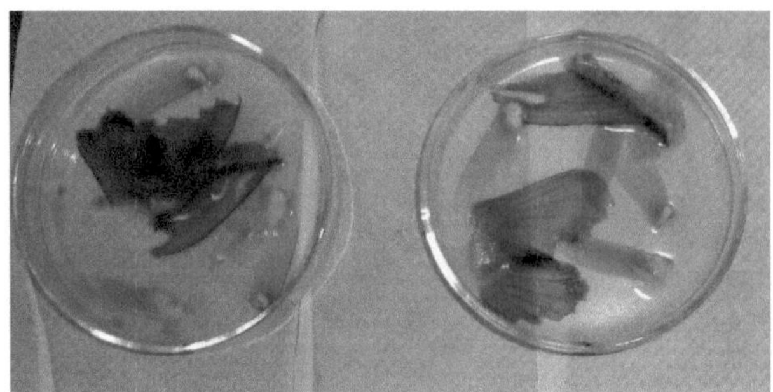

Figure 4 - Search for encysted metacercariae in fish fins.

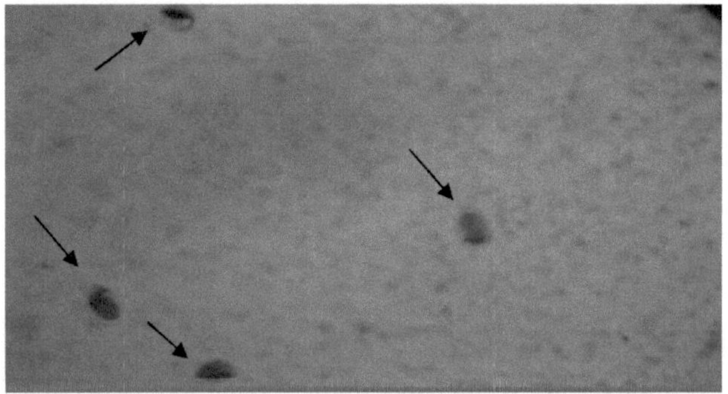

Figure 5 - Recovered metacercariae (stereoscopic microscope, 40x magnification).

CHAPTER III

Molecular diagnosis of *Taenia saginata* in the state of Tocantins.

SUMMARY

The main objective of this research was to ascertain the species-specific molecular identity of bovine cysticercus samples in the state of Tocantins. Cysticercosis was observed in cattle slaughtered in slaughterhouses in the state of Tocantins, specifically in the municipalities of Alvorada and Araguaina, located in the south and north of the state, respectively. Bovine cysticercosis is caused by *Cysticercus bovis*, the larval stage of *Taenia saginata* and once the bovine ingests the *T. saginata* egg, the *cysticercus is* ingested. *saginata egg*, the cysticercus develops and settles in different organs and systems such as the heart, lungs, liver, subcutaneous tissue, skeletal muscles, eyeballs and central nervous system, with a predilection for the striated muscles, preferably the masseter muscle, followed by the cardiac muscles and the tongue. Humans are the definitive hosts of *T. saginata* and are responsible for spreading the eggs in the environment. Teniasis is the disease caused by the adult stage of the parasite in the small intestine of humans. Cysticercosis is the disease caused by the parenteral metacestode stage in the tissues of humans and animals. Samples of live and calcified cysticercus were analyzed from March to September 2010. After DNA extraction using the phenol-chloroform method, the samples were diagnosed using the Polymerase Chain Reaction technique, using primer pairs (5'-GGCTTGTTGAATGGTTTGACG- 3') / (5'-CGACTCATGAAGATAAACAAGGT- 3') specific for *Taenia saginata*. THE average occurrence of cysticercosis during the months of collection was 0.033%. Some of the samples analyzed did not show species-specific molecular identity for *Taenia saginata*.

Keywords: *Taenia saginata,* cysticercosis, molecular biology, public health.

1 INTRODUCTION

The Phylum Platyhelminthes, Class Cestoidea, Order Cyclophyllidea and Family Taeniidae include the parasites of the genus *Taenia* spp. which has 42 species and three subspecies, 35 of which have had their life cycle completely described (LOSS-FRANK, 2000; HOBERG, 2006).

Among the parasitic diseases of veterinary medical and public health interest, bovine cysticercosis deserves to be highlighted in our country today, due to its high prevalence and the great socio-economic damage it causes (FUKUDA et al, 1998).

Bovine cysticercosis is caused by *Cysticercus bovis*, the larval stage of *T. saginata*, and once the bovine ingests the *T. saginata* egg, the *cysticercus develops, settling in different organs and systems such as the heart, lungs, liver, subcutaneous tissue and skeletal muscles. saginata egg,* the cysticercus develops and settles in different organs and systems such as the heart, lungs, liver, subcutaneous tissue, skeletal muscles, eyeballs and central nervous system, with a predilection for the striated muscles, preferably the masseter muscle, followed by the cardiac muscles and the tongue (CARVALHO et al... 2010), 2010).

The cestodes *Taenia saginata* and *Taenia solium* are responsible for human teniasis, and man is the definitive host of these parasites, which are located in the small intestine. Their larval forms (*Cysticercus bovis* and *Cysticercus cellulosae*) produce cysticercosis (URQUHART et al, 2008).

Humans contract parasitism by ingesting the larval form which is encysted in the muscle of the intermediate host, which is called a cysticercus. This infection occurs mainly through the consumption of raw or insufficiently cooked meat containing the cysticercus (URQUHART et al, 2008).

Bovine cysticercosis is not a diagnosable disease at farm level, as the animals show moderate infection with no clinical signs. The damage occurs in the final phase of beef cattle farming after slaughter, represented mainly by the condemnation of cysticercotic carcasses, causing major losses in beef exports (MONTEIRO et al , 2007). The aim of this study was to ascertain the species-specific molecular identity of bovine cysticercus samples in the state of Tocantins, as well as to carry out a differential diagnosis of cysticercosis samples using histopathology.

2 MATERIAL AND METHODS

1.1 Place of collection and laboratory analysis

The cysticercus samples used in this study were randomly collected during the *post-mortem* inspection carried out by the SIF at the slaughterhouses in Alvorada (SIF 1723 - Frigorifico Boi Brasil) and Araguaina (SIF 723 - Frigorifico Boi Forte), municipalities in the state of Tocantins, between March and September 2010. Table 1 shows the number of monthly slaughterings at each establishment and the number of cases of cysticercosis, considering live and calcified cysts.

After detecting the cysticercus, the samples were packed in plastic bags, identified and frozen, and then transported to the Veterinary Parasitology Laboratory of the School of Veterinary Medicine and Zootechny (EMVZ) of the Federal University of Tocantins (UFT), located in Araguaina - TO, where the DNA was extracted and the samples were diagnosed using the Polymerase Chain Reaction (PCR) technique.

For the species-specific molecular identification of *Taenia saginata,* the following primer pairs were used (5'-GGCTTGTTTGAATGGTTTGACG- 3') / (5-CGACTCATGAAGATAAACAAGGT- 3'). The characteristics of the primers used are described below: *Taenia saginata* COI 827 bp ; 100 bp Marker Real Biotech Cooperation, eppendorf Master cycler® ep (German) PCR-98, 1min, (94, 30sec-58, 30 sec, 72, 90 sec) X 35 cycle, 72.5 min - Taq polymerase Invitrogen.

1.2 Samples collected

The cysticercus collected were classified into two forms: live or calcified. After the *post-mortem* examination of the animals, samples were taken from the animals affected by cysticercosis in one of the aforementioned forms.

The samples were analyzed at the Veterinary Parasitology Laboratory, totaling 14 specimens. The cysticercus were thawed at room temperature, without the use of artificial means for this purpose, and then the molecular analyses were started, such as DNA extraction using the phenol-chloroform method, on the premises of the EMVZ - UFT Parasitology Laboratory, and then PCR.

Figures 1, 2 and 3 show some of the samples collected during the cysticercosis survey at the meatpacking plants mentioned above.

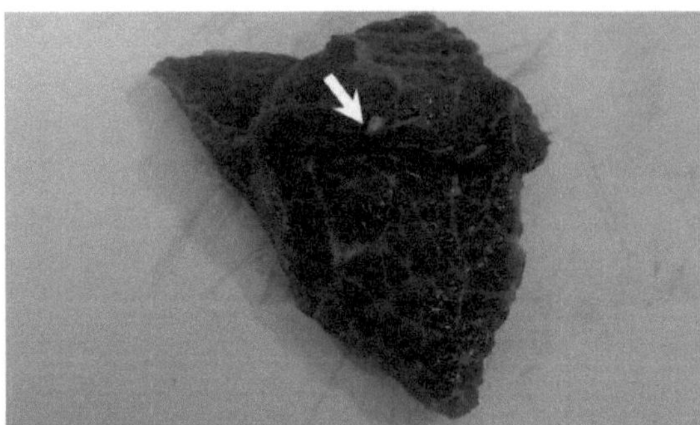

Figure 1 - Sample of masseter muscle with calcified cysticercus.

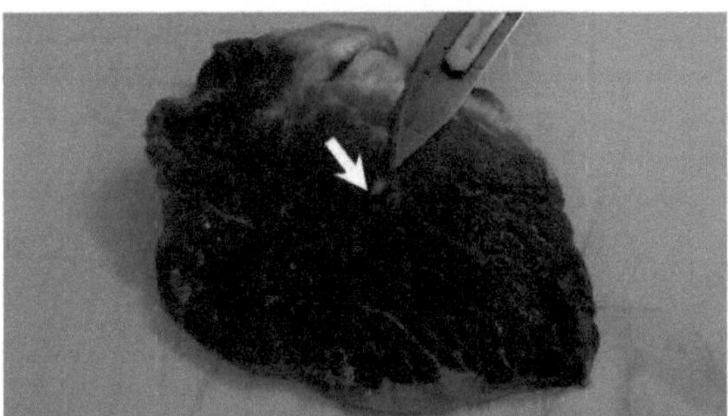

Figure 2 - Sample of masseter muscle with calcified cysticercus.

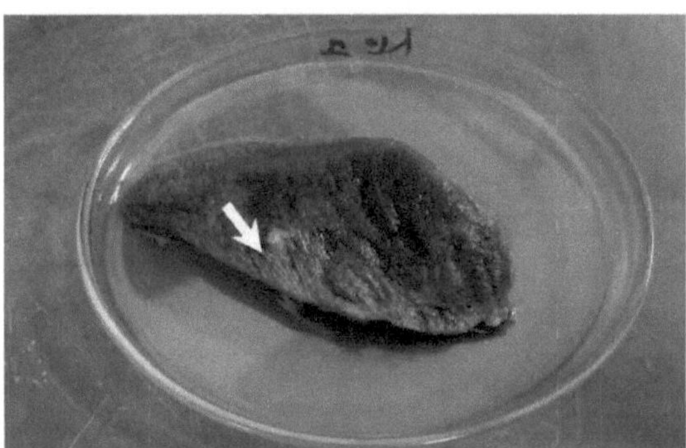

Figure 3 - Cardiac muscle sample with calcified cysticercus.

1.3 DNA extraction

To obtain DNA from the cysticercus samples, the extraction protocol based on the use of phenol-chloroform-isoamyl alcohol and ethanol precipitation was applied, as recommended by SAMBROOK et al. (1989).

Figures 4, 5, 6 and 7 show some of the equipment used to extract DNA from the samples collected.

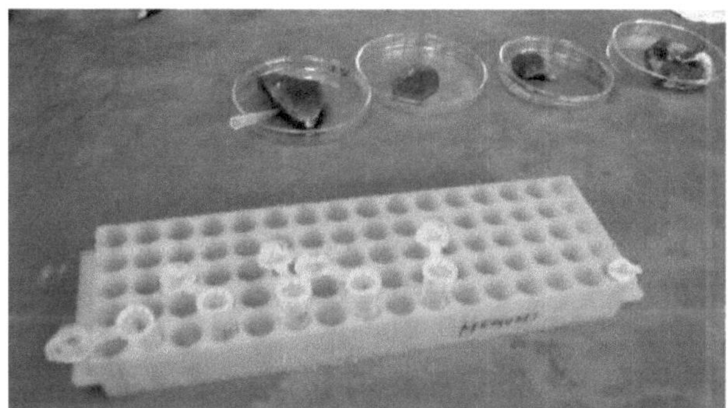

Figure 4 - Cardiac and masseter muscle samples with cysticercus for DNA extraction.

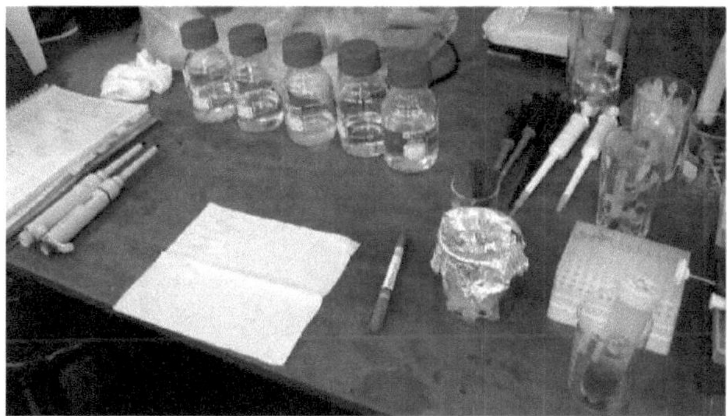

Figure 5 - Materials used for DNA extraction - Phenol-chloroform method.

3   RESULTS AND DISCUSSION

With reference to the results of the number of cases of bovine cysticercosis obtained in this study, a relatively low rate can be observed during the period from March to September 2010. The average occurrence of cysticercosis during the months of collection was low (0.033%), when compared to the work of Marques et al. (2008). These authors observed a high prevalence of bovine cysticercosis in the states of Tocantins (10.23%), São Paulo (8.76%) and Paranà (7.53%), followed by lower prevalences in the states of Minas Gerais (5.92%), Mato Grosso do Sul (4.74%), Goiàs (4.16%) and Mato Grosso (0.71%). According to SIGSIF/SISA/DDA/SFA/TO/MAPA (2011), the average occurrence of cysticercosis in the period from 01/01/2009 to 31/12/2010 in the state of Tocantins was 0.02%.

Table 1 shows the number of cattle slaughtered between March and September 2010 at the Boi Brasil and Boi Forte meatpacking plants.

Table 1 - Number of cattle slaughtered and cases of live and calcified cysticercosis (CYS) diagnosed between March and September 2010.

MONTHS	SIF 1723 *	CYS LIVE	CYS CALC.	SIF 723 **	CYS LIVE	CYS CALC.
March	8.564	01	01	15.788	03	01
April	8.811	01	02	14.863	-	04
May	8.772	02	-	13.379	-	01
June	9.270	01	01	16.050	-	06
July	7.731	02	04	18.428	02	07
August	7.998	01	03	13.754	01	03
September	7.445	01	02	13.238	01	02
TOTAL	**58.591**	**09**	**13**	**105.500**	**07**	**24**

***SIF 1723 (Frigorifico Boi Brasil) ALVORADA - TO**

****SIF 723 (Frigorifico Boi Forte) ARAGUAINA - TO** Source: SIF's 1723 and 723

The number of cases of live and calcified cysticercosis during the period of the experiment can be seen in Graphs 1 and 2. Graph 3 shows the location of the cysticercus found in the samples analyzed.

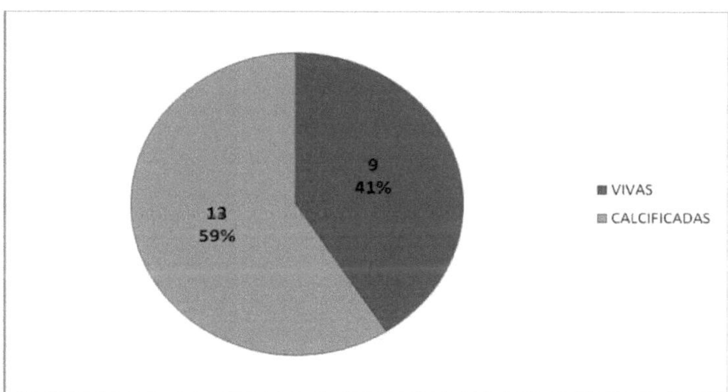

Graph 1. Number of cases of live and calcified cysticercosis from March to September 2010 (SIF - 1723).

Graph 1 shows the number of cases of live and calcified cysticercosis found at Frigorifico Boi Brasil (SIF - 1723), located in the south of the state of Tocantins, 9 and 13 cases respectively, between March and September 2010. In this establishment, a prevalence of 0.037% was obtained, with 0.015% of live samples and 0.022% of calcified samples.

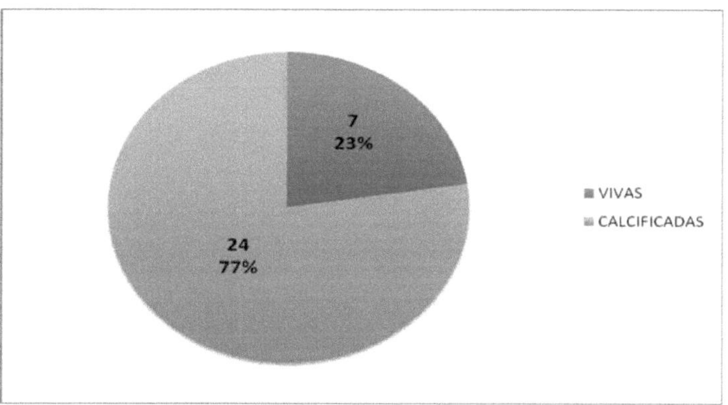

Graph 2. Number of cases of live and calcified cysticercosis from March to September 2010 (SIF - 723)

Graph 2 shows the data for Frigorifico Boi Forte (SIF - 723), located in the northern region of the state of Tocantins, where 7 cases of live cysticercosis and 24 cases of calcified cysticercus were found, giving a prevalence of 0.029% (0.006% of live samples and 0.023% of calcified samples).

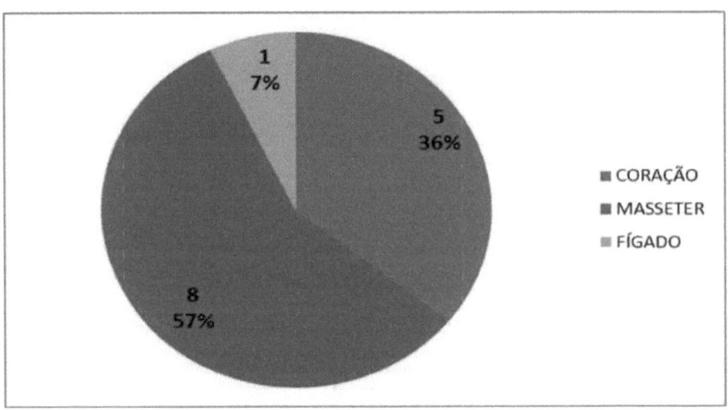

Graph 3. Location of the cysticercus found in the samples analyzed (SIF's - 723 and 1723)

The results found in this study indicate that of the 164,091 animals slaughtered, 53 were condemned for having parasitic cysts indicative of cysticercosis. However, of the 14 samples analyzed, only 8 were positive for *Taenia saginata* using the polymerase chain reaction (PCR) technique, making up 57.14% of the samples collected, as can be seen in Table 2.

Table 2 - List of cysticercus samples collected for analysis between March and September 2010.

SAMPLE NO.	CLASSIFICATION	SIF's 1723* 723**	MONTH OF COLLECTION	LOCATION/ORGANIZATION	SEX OF ANIMAL	PCR RESULT
1	Calcified	723	March	Heart	Female	Positive
2	Calcified	723	April	Heart	Female	Negative
3	Calcified	723	April	Heart	Female	Negative
4	Hooray	1723	April	Masseter	Male	Positive
5 a	Hooray	1723	July	Masseter	Female	Positive
5 b	Hooray	1723	July	Masseter	Female	Positive
1 A	Calcified	723	June	Masseter	Female	Negative
1 B	Calcified	723	June	Masseter	Female	Positive
1 C	Calcified	723	June	Masseter	Female	Negative
2	Hooray	723	August	Heart	Male	Negative
3	Calcified	1723	August	Heart	Male	Positive
4	Calcified	1723	August	Masseter	Female	Positive
5	Calcified	1723	August	Masseter	Female	Positive

6	Calcified	1723	September	Liver	Female	Negative

***SIF 1723 (Frigorifico Boi Brasil) ALVORADA - TO**

****SIF 723 (Frigorifico Boi Forte) ARAGUAINA - TO**

During this experiment, it was observed that some samples condemned as cysticercosis were not positive for this disease using the PCR technique (Figure 8). These samples were diagnosed by histopathology, which did not confirm that they were positive for cysticercosis, while some samples were positive for tuberculosis and others for hydatidosis.

Figure 6 shows the presence of giant cells, suggestive of tuberculosis. Figure 7 shows another pathology, suggestive of hydatidosis, which was detected during this study.

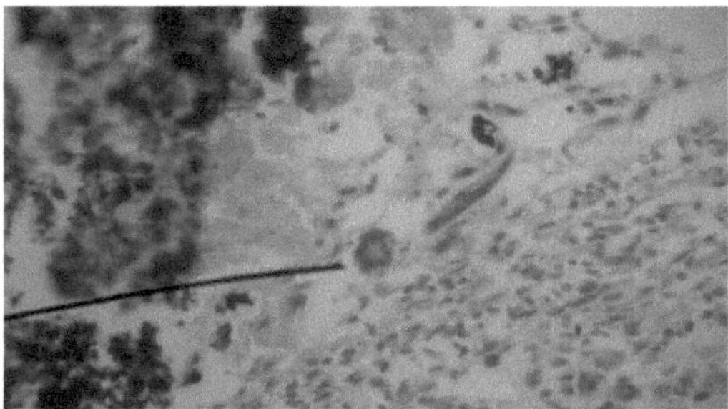

Figura 6 - Histological section of the liver, wall of a giant cell granuloma. (H.E. stain) 400x magnification.

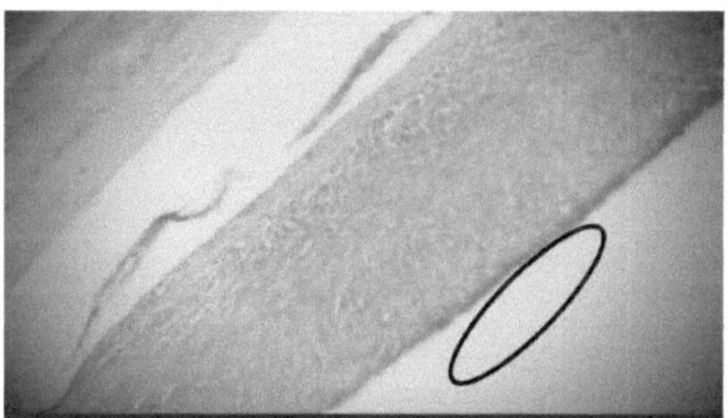

Figura 7 - Histological section of liver, absence of marking on the wall of the parasitic cyst, suggestive of hydatidosis (PAS stain) magnification 400x.

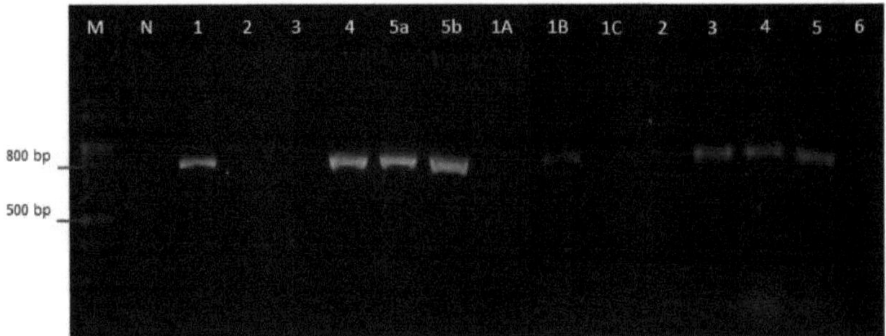

Figure 8 - 1.5% agarose gel electrophoresis specific for *Taenia saginata*.

Column M control; Column N negative; Column 1 positive sample; Columns 2 and 3 negative samples; Columns 4, 5a and 5b positive samples; Column 1A negative sample; Column 1B positive sample; Columns 1C and 2 negative samples; Columns 3, 4 and 5 positive samples; Column 6 negative sample.

4   CONCLUSIONS

•   Some of the samples analyzed did not show species-specific molecular identity to *Taenia saginata*;

•   The prevalence of bovine cysticercosis in the region studied was low, but this does not mean that basic sanitary care does not need to be taken in the face of this zoonosis;

•   Molecular diagnosis is feasible, especially when it refers to the type of pathogen in question, helping in the correct diagnosis of diseases.

5 BIBLIOGRAPHICAL REFERENCES

CARVALHO, D. A.; SATHLER, I.; ROSADO, M. **Bovine cysticercosis: learn more.** Available at: http://www.isophos.com.br/html/modules/news/article.php?storyid=143. Accessed on 10/05/2010.

FUKUDA, R. T.; SANTOS, I. F.; ANDRADE, C. R. Comparative study of the diaphragm inspection technique for the diagnosis of bovine cysticercosis. **Food Hygiene.** v.12, n° 55, p.51-62, 1998.

HOBERG, E.P. Phylogeny of *Taenia* : species definitions origins of human parasites. **Parasitology International,** v. 55, S23 - S30, 2006.

LOSS-FRANK, B. An update of Verstefs (1969). "Taxonomic revision of the genus *Taenia* Linnaeus" (Cestoda) in table format. **Systematic Parasitology,** v.45, n.1, p.155-183, 2000.

MARQUES, G.M.; BUZI, K.A.; GALINDO, L.A.; BALDINI, E.D.; BIONDI, G.F. Evaluation of cysticercosis condemnation records in cattle slaughtered in meatpacking plants in the central-western region of the state of São Paulo - 1996 to 2000.

Veterinària e Zootecnia, v.15, n.1, p.114-120, 2008.

MONTEIRO, L. L.; PINTO, P. S. A.; SALCEDO, J. H. P.; ARAÙJO, J. V.; SANTOS, W. L. M.; CECON, P. R. *Taenia solium* larval antigens in ELISA for the diagnosis of bovine cysticercosis. **Arquivo Brasileiro de Medicina Veterinària e Zootecnia.** v.59, n.1, p.21-25, 2007.

SAMBROOK, J.; FRITSCH, E.F.; MANIATIS, T. *Molecular Cloning. A Laboratory Manual.* 2nd ed. Cold Spring Harbor: Cold Spring Harbor Laboratory Press, 1989.

SIGSIF/SISA/DDA/SFA/TO/MAPA - Sistema de Informaçôes Gerenciais do Serviço de Inspeçâo Federal/Serviço de Inspeçâo e Saùde Animal/Departamento de Defesa Animal/Superintendência Federal de Agricultura do Estado do Tocantins/Ministério da Agricultura, Pecuària e Abastecimento. 2011.

URQUHART, G.M.; ARMOUR, J.; DUNCAN, J.L.; DUNN, A.M.; JENNINGS, F.W. **Parasitologia veterinària** 2 ed. p.89 Rio de Janeiro: Guanabara Koogan, 2008.

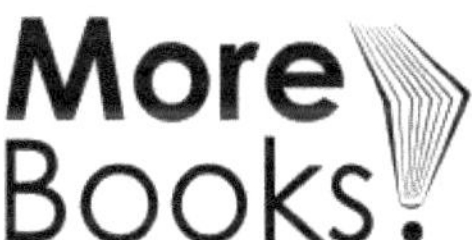

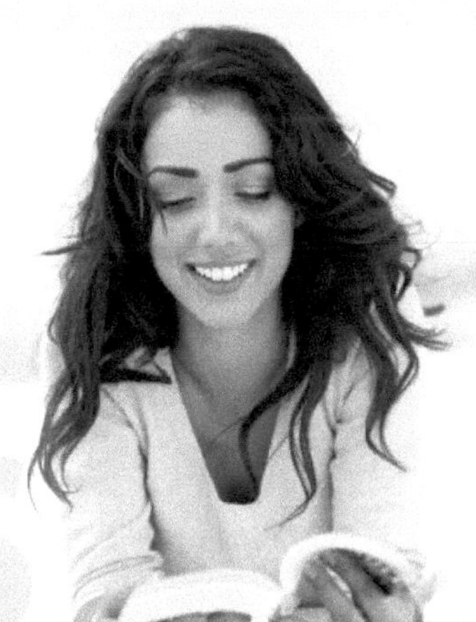

I want morebooks!

Buy your books fast and straightforward online - at one of world's fastest growing online book stores! Environmentally sound due to Print-on-Demand technologies.

Buy your books online at
www.morebooks.shop

Kaufen Sie Ihre Bücher schnell und unkompliziert online – auf einer der am schnellsten wachsenden Buchhandelsplattformen weltweit! Dank Print-On-Demand umwelt- und ressourcenschonend produzi ert.

Bücher schneller online kaufen
www.morebooks.shop

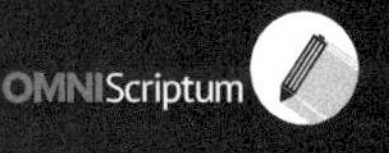